IMPOTENCE
Physiological, Psychological, Surgical Diagnosis and Treatment

PERSPECTIVES IN SEXUALITY
Behavior, Research, and Therapy

Series Editor: RICHARD GREEN
State University of New York at Stony Brook

NEW DIRECTIONS IN SEX RESEARCH
Edited by Eli A. Rubinstein, Richard Green, and Edward Brecher

PROGRESS IN SEXOLOGY
Edited by Robert Gemme and Connie Christine Wheeler

HANDBOOK OF SEX THERAPY
Edited by Joseph LoPiccolo and Leslie LoPiccolo

THE PREVENTION OF SEXUAL DISORDERS: Issues and Approaches
Edited by C. Brandon Qualls, John P. Wincze, and David H. Barlow

IMPOTENCE: Physiological, Psychological, Surgical Diagnosis and Treatment
Gorm Wagner and Richard Green

SEX EDUCATION IN THE EIGHTIES: The Challenge of Healthy Sexual Evolution
Edited by Lorna Brown

IMPOTENCE
Physiological, Psychological, Surgical Diagnosis and Treatment

Gorm Wagner, M.D.
University of Copenhagen
Copenhagen, Denmark

and

Richard Green, M.D.
State University of New York
Stony Brook, New York

PLENUM PRESS • NEW YORK AND LONDON

Library of Congress Cataloging in Publication Data

Wagner, Gorm.
Impotence : physiological, psychological, surgical diagnosis and treatment.

(Perspectives in sexuality)
Bibliography: p.
Includes index.
1. Impotence. 2. Impotence—Psychosomatic aspects. I. Green, Richard, 1936- . II. Title. III. Series. [DNLM: 1. Impotence—Diagnosis. 2. Impotence—Therapy. WJ 709 W133i]
RC889.W24 616.692 81-15688
ISBN 0-306-40719-1 AACR2

Wilhelm Reich was a pioneer in the study of the physiology of human sexuality. In 1942, having fled Germany for Denmark, Reich privately published a monograph on the function of the orgasm. Reproduced on the cover of this book are four of his original recordings from that historic work.

Printed in the United States of America

To the sexually functional men
who helped give us life

KAI H. WAGNER

and

LEO H. GREEN

Preface

Impotence. The word strikes at the bedrock of a man's worth. Its implications far exceed the inability to have a penile erection. The man is without power—ineffectual. Ancient statues represented with an oversized erect penis attest to the historic conscious meaning of the phallus. Magnificent spires, memorial monuments, and the awe generated by the sight of rockets and missiles attest to the unconscious meaning.

At the medical-superstitious level, men have invoked countless strategies for improving or restoring potency. They have included ritualistic dances, concoctions, and mechanical aids. Some survive to the present.

More recently, verbal therapies have taken their place, ranging from simple exhortation to the uncovering of complex unconscious symbolic conflicts. Other therapies borrow from theories of learning, based on experiments with mice and men.

The growth of modern endocrinology, with the isolation of "sex steroids," heralded another treatment strategy: hormones. Later, engineers entered with surgically implantable mechanical devices. And, most recently, the technology of microsurgery has offered the possibility of physiological restoration of a compromised vascular supply, a necessary component of erection.

This complex of treatment strategies clearly divides into two major categories: the psychogenic and the organic. As elsewhere, such mind–body dualism ignores the vital role of the interaction between mind and body. While there are persons for whom erection is impossible by purely psychic means because of interruption of neurogenic and vascular architecture, and other persons with a mechanically intact system, also incapable of erection, ignoring mind–body interaction is perilous. It is in this gray area, where differential diagnosis engages the relative weights of organic versus psychogenic elements, that much investigatory excitement exists.

These recent developments inspired us to write this book. Whenever a field enters a new growth phase of knowledge, there is an inevitable lag between scattered innovative journal publications and the integration of new knowledge into a comprehensive text. This book serves that function and goes beyond. It also includes previously unpublished research.

Perhaps with this newest era in the understanding, diagnosis, and treatment of *erectile dysfunction* or *erectile failure* (less pejorative terms than *impotence*), scientism will replace superstition regarding a bodily function that is integral to a man's self-image, conducive to great sensual pleasure, and necessary for survival of the species. This encompassing triad, this unique set of human dimensions, merits no less.

Although both of the principal authors contributed to all chapters, where one author assumed primary responsibility, he is cited as sole author. We emphasize, however, that this book is a joint endeavor.

Illustrations were drawn by Ulla Bang Lundblad, Skodsborg, Denmark. For typing various parts of the manuscript, sorting references and keeping track of correspondence, we are grateful to Ulla Brat, Anne Boesen, Vibeke Brabrand, Alice Schou, and Merete Lassen, of Copenhagen, and Virginia Bentley and Carol Sancimo, of Stony Brook.

Parts of the research presented were made possible by grants from the NOVO Fund, Copenhagen, and the Danish Medical Research Council (SLF-512-20488).

RICHARD GREEN, M.D.
GORM WAGNER, M.D.

Contents

Case Vignettes

Presenting Syndromes

The following case vignettes offer a representative, heterogeneous sampling of men presenting with conditions of erectile failure. The material in the subsequent chapters should enable the reader to formulate a program for diagnosis and clinical management. At the book's end, the diagnostic and management procedures that were followed with each patient are described, along with clinical outcome.[1]

A-1 Case Vignette

A 47-year-old married worker with satisfactory work and financial conditions was referred by his family physician for treatment of erectile dysfunction. Apart from a nonspecific urethritis 15 years earlier, he had no history of medical problems.

His earlier sexual life had included masturbation since teenage, initial sexual intercourse at 20, and four premarital relationships. He married at 25, his wife being 20.

They have three children, ages 20, 16, and 12. After an initially satisfactory erection pattern, sexual problems began six years ago. In the beginning, he had problems maintaining an erection and a tendency toward premature ejaculation. The erectile failure progressed gradually, and, during the past six years, he has not been able to obtain a full erection either with his wife, during masturbation, or with another woman with whom he "tested" his erectile capability.

Morning erections have ceased and current erections are of modest degree. Sex drive has not diminished. He had visited his physician several times with the

[1]Each patient is identified by a letter. The sequence of case histories at the book's beginning and end remain the same. A-1 refers to the presenting syndrome. A-2 refers to the same patient's diagnosis, clinical management, and outcome.

same complaint. For a period of three months, he was treated with methyltestosterone without effect. The patient had talked openly with his wife about the problem and had earlier believed that she was understanding. Nevertheless, on several occasions, she accused him of having a mistress and of no longer being interested in her. He denied her claims and stated that he is afraid of failure if she initiates love play.

Four years ago, the patient had a two-year period of alcohol abuse. At that time, his work was very stressing. He recovered by changing his work pattern and now drinks only occasionally.

B-1 Case Vignette

A 33-year-old salesman was referred by a gynecologist for erectile dysfunction. He had been through two years of infertility investigations with his 32-year-old wife. Erectile ability had declined gradually during the previous 14 months. He has two brothers who both have children. His marriage is of 6 years' duration, and he had previously been living with another woman who used contraceptives. He described no economic problems. He smokes and drinks modestly.

The first sign of erectile dysfunction occurred "on the Saturday before Easter the year before." The couple had been told to spend that time together, to relax, and to have an active sexual life because of anticipated ovulation. They drank half a bottle of wine, and during an attempt at intercourse, he was unable to erect. The next day, he managed to get a semierection with vaginal intromission.

The rigidity problem has worsened, and he is obtaining no tumescence with sexual stimulation. Morning erections have become fewer, but there is still some stiffness. His wife discourages intercourse in the morning. He visited his former girlfriend, with whom he always had a well-functioning sex life. However, he was unable to erect in their attempt at intercourse, and she ridiculed him.

He states that he wants a penile prosthesis.

C-1 Case Vignette

A 35-year-old man was referred from the social authorities for treatment of alcoholism. His parents divorced when he was 12, and for some months, he lived in institutions. Later, he returned to living with his mother and his two younger sisters. He attended school for eight years and is a skilled technical factory worker. During the last two years, he has not been at his usual work but has worked intermittently as a bartender. He is married to a 34-year-old woman with a part-time job. There are two children, aged 4 and 8 years. Their economic situation is rather insecure.

He usually has severe gastritis during drinking periods. His liver was found to be slightly affected during a routine checkup by his general practitioner. He had been in a hospital once for a head injury that occurred during inebriation. He has a slight paresthesia in both legs. He was hospitalized for one night in a psychiatric ward because of drinking. The following morning he demanded to leave the hospital. He denied any psychiatric complications apart from a slight reduction in short-term memory.

He first became inebriated at age 15. Since age 19, he has been drinking alcohol (mostly beer) in excess. During the last three years, he has shown signs of the alcohol dependence syndrome (e.g., physical withdrawal, morning drinking, critical point of no return, daily alcohol intake, and blackouts). He drinks about 20 bottles of beer a day.

He came for treatment at the insistence of social authorities who had refused to offer him any kind of economic help if he continued drinking. At the first visit, he was rather abstinence-marked and confused, but he agreed to start treatment with disulfiram (Antabuse®). For the first week, he was supplied with chlordiazepoxide (Librium®) in doses of 150 mg a day, then reduced to 15 mg a day. From the second week, he was given neuroleptic treatment, chlorprotixen (Truxal®) 45 mg a day.

Four weeks later, when he had attended the clinic, he explained that he had become impotent. He believed that Antabuse® was the main reason for the erectile failure, and he wanted to discontinue this treatment. He argued that he had never had sexual problems before and that if he had to become impotent from this treatment, he would prefer drinking.

D-1 Case Vignette

A 39-year-old engineer was referred with a history of six months' erectile problems. During this period, he had not been able to experience intercourse in the superior position. While he experienced a full, rigid erection during foreplay, soon after vaginal intromission the stiffness disappeared when coital movements were initiated. Quite often he experienced pain in the gluteal muscles during coitus. This pain interrupted intercourse. Sometimes his erection reappeared. He also noticed the ability to maintain intravaginal erection when lying in a lateral position and avoiding activity.

He had been married to his present wife five years, beginning one year following a previous eight-year marriage with two children. His present marriage is childless, as both partners are hard working and enjoying an active social life. They have intercourse every night. He described their relationship as being on a high intellectual and emotional level, with great mutual concern. Morning erections are unaltered. He had read of psychogenic erectile dysfunction but had not been able to find any similarities to his own situation. His wife is very understanding and has done "everything" to make the best of the situation.

He feels no other somatic inadequacies except that during the last year he has experienced extreme weakness in the legs during and after walking.

E-1 Case Vignette

A 34-year-old diabetic male complained of erectile dysfunction at a regular checkup in an outpatient clinic. Diabetes had been diagnosed 15 years earlier, and since then, he has been taking insulin. Metabolic regulation is average to poor. His present treatment is 40 international units of intermediate-acting insulin in the morning and a diet of 2600 cal per day. He does not smoke and has no daily intake of alcohol. He has been married for 10 years and has two children, ages 3 and 8. The marriage is described as harmonic. Their social and economic situation is stable.

Erectile dysfunction had developed insidiously over the prior two years, and coitus has become impossible. There are no morning erections. Masturbation is possible with ejaculation and relief of sexual tension.

Laboratory data: 24-hr glucose excretion was 95 g, with urine positive for ketone bodies. Serum creatinine was 115 μmol/1, with urine positive for albumin. Ophthalmoscopy showed proliferative retinopathy.

The patient's interest in sexual activity has remained unaltered, but he now tries to avoid sexual contact in order not to fail. The couple have not discussed the problem between themselves, and he assumes that his wife must be suffering from his condition. He has tried to have intercourse twice with other women, once with an attractive woman from work and once with a prostitute. During the second of these occasions, he obtained good tumescence, but no stiffness.

F-1 Case Vignette

A 19-year-old shop assistant was referred from his family physician as he had been unable to perform vaginal coitus with his 20-year-old girlfriend. They had tried 16 times without success.

He had an uneventful childhood with a younger brother, a pleasant and understanding mother, and a kind father. However, the family never talked about sex. He received some sexual information at school but was not very interested.

At age 14, he noticed that his penis did not look like those of other boys when sexually stimulated. In pornography magazines, he observed the same difference. At age 16, he went to his family physician, who told him not to bother and said that it would work adequately when the time "was ripe." During the next years, he went to several libraries and read about erection and erection failure, and he read that failure could only be for psychic reasons. However, he refused to believe that he had a psychic disorder that prevented him from having a normal erection.

After having met a girl with whom he fell in love, and still not being able to erect, he felt very insecure. His girlfriend went to his mother and told her about the situation. The mother and the patient went to the family physician, who referred him to a plastic surgeon.

G-1 Case Vignette

A 48-year-old teacher married to a 46-year-old asthmatic woman was referred because two years earlier he had suddenly lost his ability to have a penile erection. He had grown up in a devoutly religious home where there was no talk of sex. He had always been shy and a hard worker. He married a colleague at age 34.

Because of his wife's disease, he had not asked for medical help earlier, but he now feels that if he is to have anything done, it should be before he grows too old. There has been no demand from his wife during the last two to three years, although she has recovered somewhat from her illness.

He had been seen by his family physician, who suggested psychotherapy, which he refused, and by a urologist, who performed a cavernosogram that was normal.

H-1 Case Vignette

A 24-year-old unmarried ski instructor reported never having been able to obtain a full erection during sexual arousal. He had been brought up in a wealthy family with strict social guidelines but a relaxed attitude toward religion. His parents were caring but professionally engaged.

His first masturbation experience was at 14, and his first attempt at intercourse at 21. While he was able to effect vaginal intromission, the penis did not really become hard. This caused him considerable anxiety.

He was seen by his family physician and examined for diseases related to erectile dysfunction, including diabetes, neuropathy, and endocrine disorders. He was then sent to a neurologist, who could not find any pathology by cystometry, examination of genital reflexes, EEG, or general examination. Referral was then made to a psychologist, who treated him for eight months without improvement.

I-1 Case Vignette

A 62-year-old man had been unable to have a full erection for vaginal intromission for 2½ years. He has been married for 35 years to a woman 5 years younger than he. There are four adult children and three grandchildren. He had run his own business and did well for many years but suffered an economic collapse five years ago. His wife began to work and built her own successful business. His business has now recovered and is in good financial condition. He reports good intellectual companionship with his wife.

Coitus is attempted one or two times a month. He usually has to stop because of lack of erection. He feels a great need for physical love but has had no extramarital relationships.

The patient has suggested that he may have a physical block of blood flow and has requested reconstructive surgery.

CHAPTER 1

Erection

Anatomy

GORM WAGNER

The penis serves three major functions. It serves as the male sex organ during coitus. It leads urine from the bladder to the surface of the body via the urethra. And, as the seminal vesicles open into the urethra, it is a pathway for sperm and spermatic fluid to collect in the urethra before expulsion as an ejaculate.

The penis is chiefly composed of cavernous (erectile) and spongiose tissue. When flaccid, only narrow spaces exist. Engorgement of the cavernous tissue with blood gives rise to a considerable increase in size (tumescence) and may culminate in full erection.

The size of the free, mobile part of the flaccid penis varies. In a pioneering study of 50 men aged 18–53 years (mean age, 26.6 years) attending a venereal clinic in Munich, the length and circumference of the penis was measured (Loeb, 1899). The length was 9.4 cm ± 0.15 (mean ± SEM). The calculated diameter from these values was 28.8 mm ± 0.3, and the volume was 62 ml ± 1.7, with a range from 36.9 to 87.5 ml. Figure 1 shows the closer relation between volume and circumference than between volume and length and depicts the spread of circumference to a given length and vice versa. It is clearly seen that there is no correlation between the circumference and the length of the flaccid penis.

This material, now more than 80 years old, seems to be the only large body of published material with objectively performed measurements. Masters and Johnson (1966) have not published the figures from their sample but have discussed the change during erection in two selected groups. From a study of 312 men, they found evidence to support the statement of Piesol (1907) that the size of the penis has a less constant relation to general physical development than that of any other organ.

The only large-scale study of penile length and circumference is of subjec-

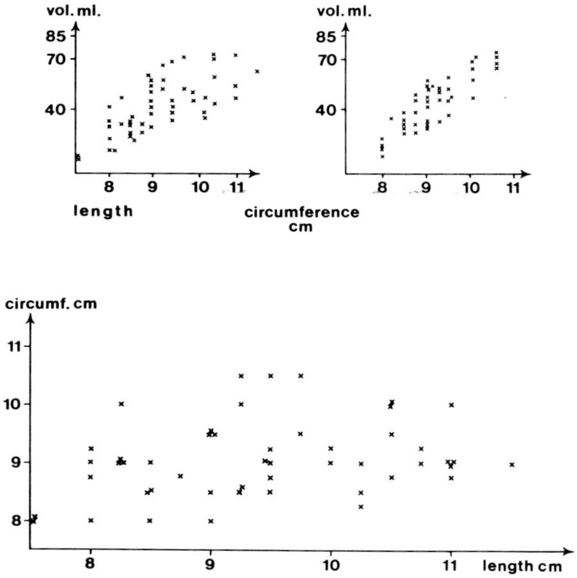

Figure 1. Objective penile measures in the flaccid state from 50 men between 18 and 53 years of age. The calculated volume is in relation to length (upper left) and circumference (upper right). The circumference gives a better indication of volume. There is no correlation between circumference and length (bottom). (Calculated and modified after Loeb, 1899.)

tively reported data and represents 2,310 white men. This study was recently published in some detail in the newer Kinsey data (Gebhard and Johnson, 1979). Figure 15 (Chapter 2) gives these measurements in diagrammatic form. It will be noted that the means of these measures are in good agreement with the values given by Loeb. Exact comparison cannot be made as the American organs were to be measured to the "nearest quarter inch," but the respondents were not able to do so and mainly grouped themselves according to the nearest half inch.

Structure

In the standing man, the penis hangs down, with its ventral (urethral) surface in close apposition to the anterior surface of the scrotum, as shown in the sagittal section in Figure 2. Traditionally, three cylinders are described as the main structures of the organ. Two are a set, the paired cavernous bodies (corpora cavernosa penis) that constitute the dorsal and lateral part of the penis. Functionally, however, they are a unit and were originally described as such by the Dutch anatomist de Graaf in the seventeenth century. The third cylinder is the smaller, unpaired spongiose body (the corpus spongiosum penis) that is traversed by the urethra.

In the shaft, the corpus penis and the cavernous bodies present as a flattened dorsal surface with a slight longitudinal groove in the middle where they earlier fused. The lateral surfaces are rounded, and on the urethral face, a furrow is present, giving space for the spongiose body. Figure 3 shows the relationship of the structures. At the distal end of the organ, the corpus spongiosum expands into the cone-shaped end, the glans. Before circumcision, it is covered by the foreskin, the preputium (prepuce), and the skin. After circumcision, it presents partly or completely uncovered. On the tip of the glans, the urethra ends with a vertical slit opening, the external urethral orifice. The base of the glans is excavated and, like a hood, covers the anterior conically shaped part of the united cavernous bodies (Figures 2 and 3). The margin of the glans and the corona projects beyond the end of the corpora cavernosa toward the root of the penis.

The skin of the shaft is thin, loosely bound, and pigmented on the urethral surface along the median raphe, which is continuous with the raphe of the scrotum. The skin covering the peripheral part is without hair; at the root, sparse pubic hair may occur. There are sweat glands and—especially on the lateral and urethral surfaces—sebaceous glands. The skin continues into the free fold of the prepuce overlapping the glans. It is bound to the sulcus coronarius and continues, now firmly bound, around the corona and covers the entire glans. On the urethral face, a small median fold, the frenulum of the prepuce, is connected to the deep

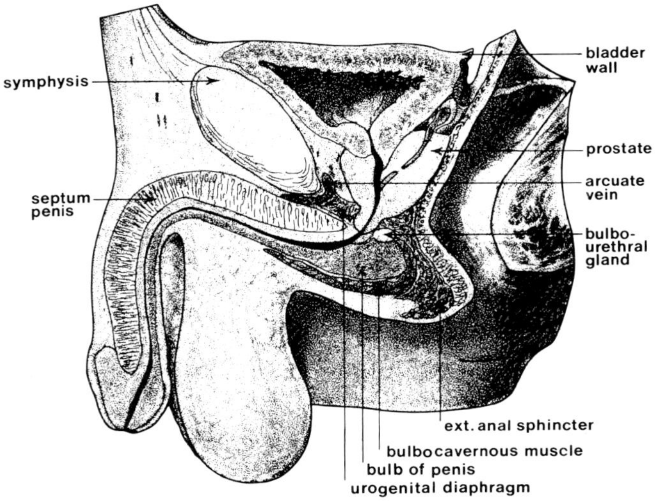

Figure 2. Midline sagittal section of the male pelvis presenting structures in relation to the penis.

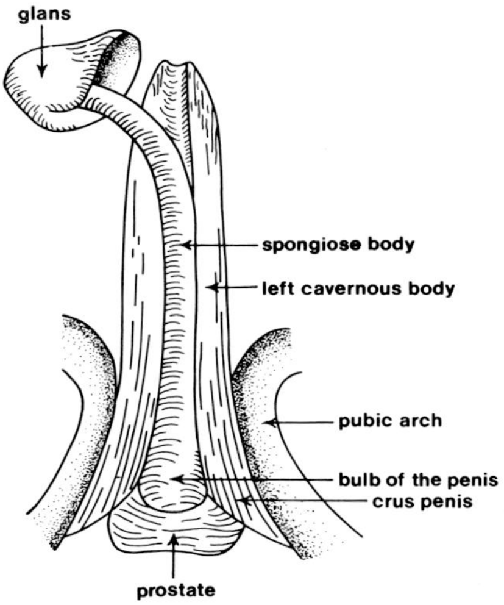

Figure 3. Drawing from an anatomical preparation and viewed from below showing the two main structures of which the penis is composed. The right and left cavernous bodies are encapsulated by a thick fibrous sheath and form a unity. Inside this structure, the pressure is built up to make the penis rigid. The glans and the spongiose body form another unity encapsulated together. This structure never achieves a pressure as high as that inside the cavernous bodies during sexual arousal.

part of the prepuce. The appearance of the skin on the glans is more of a mucous membrane, and the color varies from light red to violet.

At the root of the penis, the three corpora separate. The cavernous bodies diverge sideways, and, gradually tapering, each becomes intimately attached by fibrous tissue to the periosteum of the pubic arch (Figure 3). Each crus is covered by the ischiocavernous muscle. The corpus spongiosum lies under and between the cavernous bodies and becomes enlarged, forming the globular mass called the *bulbus penis*. This structure is covered by the bulbocavernous muscle. Neither of these striated muscles is involved in erection in man but contracts rhythmically during ejaculation, helping the antegrade propulsion of semen. The penis is thus firmly fixed at its root by fibrous tissue as well as by muscles and is further bound to the above-lying anterior surface of the pubic symphysis by two ligaments. The deep-lying suspensory ligament of the penis is a fibrous structure fanning toward and attaching broadly to the fibrous sheath encapsulating the cavernous bodies. The more elastic fundiform ligament extends downward from the abdominal wall and loops around the penis, interspersing the superficial penile fascia. This fascial sheath is mostly composed of smooth muscle fibers and elastic fibers and continues into the tunica dartos of the scrotum. Deep to the superficial fascia is found the deep fascia of the penis (Buck's fascia), which is thin but tight, consisting of elastic fibers. It is fixed to the base of the glans and forms a common envelope for the spongiose and cavernous bodies. It partly gives insertion to the fibers of the ischiocavernosus and bulbocavernosus muscles and at the root of the penis is tightly connected with the attachment to the bone. Although it is bound to the tunica albuginea of the cavernous bodies, it provides space for vessels and nerves running between these sheaths.

The cavernous bodies, the major erectile organs of the penis, are enclosed in a thick, dense fibrous capsule, the tunica albuginea, measuring 2–4 mm in thickness in the flaccid state. It contains some elastic fibers as well. From this capsule, the septum is formed in the median. Figure 4 demonstrates the configuration of the cavernous bodies in cross-section. The septum is highly incomplete in a large part of the mobile part of the penis but becomes more complete before the cavernous bodies diverge into their crura (Forster, 1903). Some mammals have a bone formation developed in the septum, called the *os penis*.

Anchored on the inside of the tunica and running transversely and slightly obliquely are cylindrical strands of fibrous tissue. These hang loosely in the cavernous tissue in the flaccid state. They are probably identical with the trabeculae described from microscopic sections by the older anatomists. The strands differ from the major part of the cavernous tissue by their whitish color and organized orientation. The structural relationship of the fibrous tissues, the tunica albuginea, the septum, and the strands is responsible for the modest compliance and the preservation of the principle outline of the cavernous bodies whether flaccid or erect.

The cavernous tissue is built like a sponge, with irregular strands dominated by smooth muscle cells. The cells intermingle and are fixed to each other as well as to the scarce connective tissue. The tissue contains capillaries and nerves as well and is lined by endothelial cells on the part facing the interstices. The distance

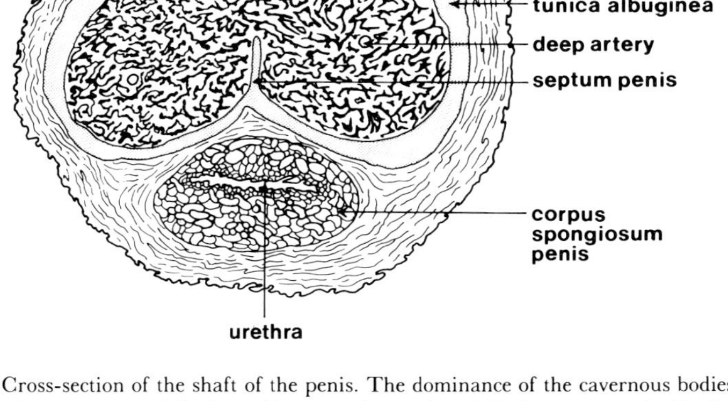

Figure 4. Cross-section of the shaft of the penis. The dominance of the cavernous bodies is shown. The trabecular tissue is mainly formed by smooth muscle, while the structure inside the spongiose body is dominated by elastic tissue. In this preparation, only the deep dorsal vessels are clearly shown.

between the walls of a caverna may vary from the larger central to the smaller peripheral but is estimated to be around 1 mm in the flaccid state to 6 mm in the erect state. The cavernous smooth musculature, which is the quantitatively dominating structure of the cavernous body, is fixed on the inside of the tunica albuginea. Only a small amount of intermingling of cells is noticed on the interface site.

The corpus spongiosum is encapsulated in its own tunica albuginea, which is thinner and contains less fibrous and more elastic fibers than that of the cavernous bodies. The tissue of the bulbar and the urethral part of the corpus spongiosum is also built as a framework with interstices, more regular than that of the cavernous body, but with much fewer smooth muscle cells, and is abundantly supplied with elastic fibers. This architecture makes it ideal for giving passage to fluid in the urethra and closing off as soon as the fluid has passed. The buildup of a "pressure chamber," as suggested by Marberger (1974), would be facilitated by this kind of structure. During the first phase of the ejaculation—that is, the internal emission of semen from the seminal ducts, the vesicles, and the prostate—the fluid can ben seen collecting and undulating in the bulbar part of the urethra a few seconds before the external ejaculation (Wagner, 1976).

The glans is built up differently from the rest of the erectile tissues. Covered with very thin and firmly adherent skin, it has no fibrous sheath but contains much fibrous connective tissue. The spongelike appearance is due to a rich venous plexus with numerous anastomoses. The veins are characterized by very thick muscular walls.

It should be understood that the structural differences among the glans, the cavernous body, and the urethral and bulbar part of the spongiose body are the basis for their functional difference and their participation in erection and ejaculation.

The Blood Supply

Recent descriptions of disorders in the vascular system leading to and from the penis and causing erectile dysfunction have led to increased interest in the arterial supply of the penis. The abdominal aorta divides into the two common iliac arteries. From each of these, the internal iliac or hypogastric artery derives and continues as the internal pudendal artery after giving off large branches to the gluteal muscles (Figure 5). After giving off the perineal artery, the vessel is called the *penile artery* and runs horizontally, piercing the urogenital diaphragm. The most extensive study of the branching of the penile artery is the dissection material of Forster (1903). Generally, there are three major branches: the bulbosa or urethral artery, the deep artery, and the dorsal artery, each of them paired. The interindividual variability of their branching, where they pierce the tunica

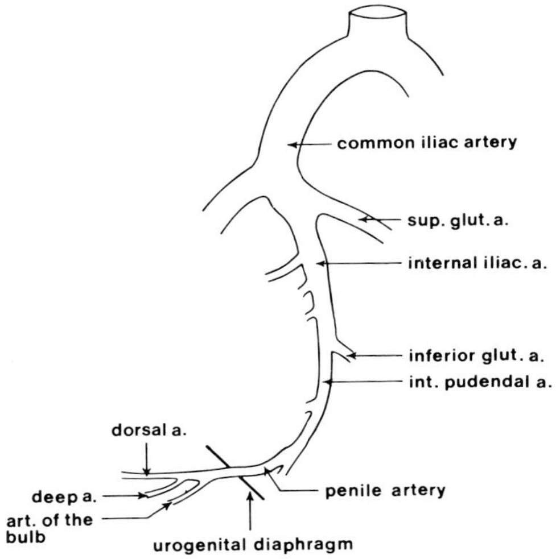

Figure 5. A schematic presentation of the arterial vessels maintaining the blood supply to the penis. The term *penile artery* is not used by all anatomists. The dorsal artery and the deep artery are the two important arteries in the development and the maintenance of erection.

albuginea and how they intercommunicate, is great. A common course of the bulbourethral arteries is to anastomose and then diverge and pierce the bulb of the spongiose body running anterior in the spongiose tissue and to some extent communicating with the cavernous bodies.

The dorsal arteries seem in their course to be the most constant in running on each side of the unpaired large dorsal vein (Figure 4) deep to Buck's fascia. Branches are sent off running obliquely forward around the cavernous bodies, partly piercing the tunica albuginea, and partly giving branches to the spongiose tissue.

The glans receives its main arterial supply from the dorsal artery. The fascia and skin of the penis receive blood partly from the dorsal artery and partly from external pudendal arteries.

The main arterial supply of the erectile tissue of the cavernous bodies is the paired deep artery entering the tissue central to the point where the two crura merge. It can be followed almost to the tip of the erectile body and gives branches to the cavernous tissue. Many anastomoses are found between the arteries.

Evidence of the abundance of arteriovenous (A-V) shunts on all levels of the arterial branching has been accumulating for more than a century, mainly through the work of Central European anatomists like Müller (1840), Langer (1862), Kiss (1921), Stieve (1930), Watzka (1936), Rotter and Schürmann (1950), Conti (1952, 1953), and Clara (1956). The A-V anastomoses occur outside as well as inside the tunica albuginea. Figure 6 is a photo that demonstrates one of these direct communications from the dorsal artery to a branch of the dorsal vein. This is only one type outside the fibrous tissue arising from the larger arterial branches. They are reported to have an inner diameter of 100 μ (Newman, *et al.*, 1964). Another type of anastomosis, presumably A-V, has been found running from the central artery to the vessels in parallel on the dorsal surface of the spongiose body (Wagner, Willis, and Rasmussen, unpublished).

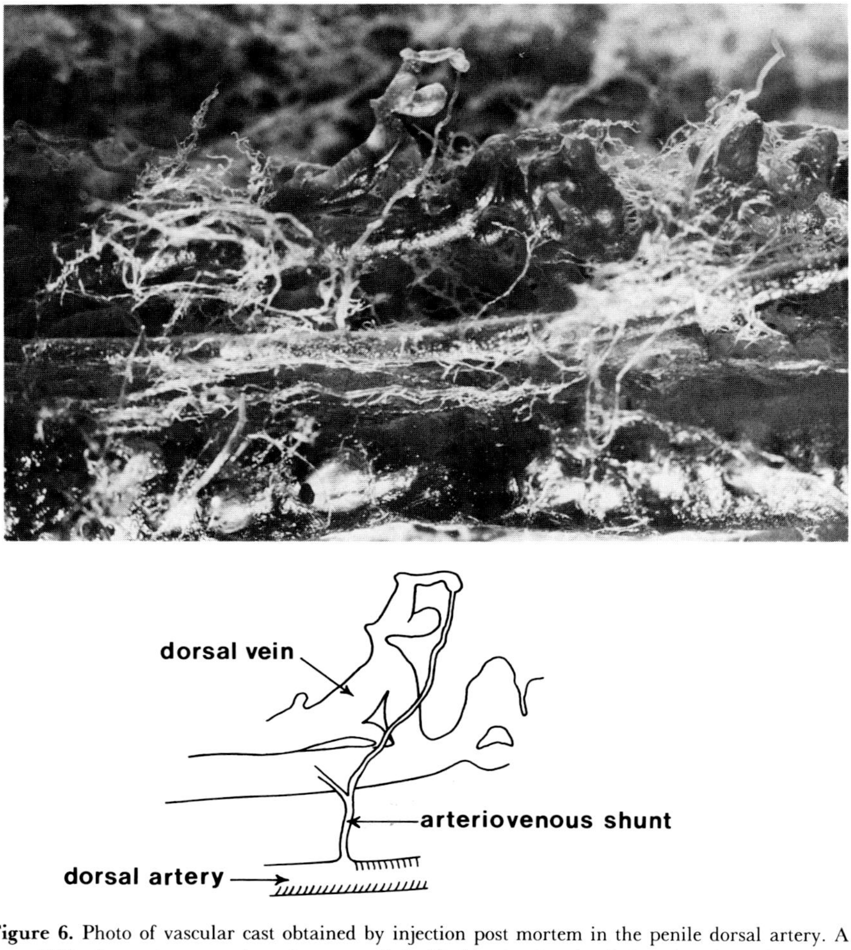

Figure 6. Photo of vascular cast obtained by injection post mortem in the penile dorsal artery. A large (100-μ) arteriovenous shunt is seen and clarified in the drawing below the photo. Only few direct connections between the arterial and venous systems are found in the dorsal space outside the tunica albuginea. All the material seen in the photo fills the vascular bed.

A predominant type in the cavernous tissue is the epithelioid arteriovenous anastomosis (Figure 7), originally described by Müller (1840) but denied for decades by later researchers. After piercing the tunica albuginea, the arterial branches have a tortuous course (helicine arteries), are almost curled up, and (1) give off branches opening directly into the cavernous tissue; (2) divide into capillaries, most of which are within the smooth-muscle framework; and (3) give off short vessels that have direct communication with the outlet ("venous") system. "Helicinous arteries" is a proper description of the appearance in the flaccid state. Most of the intracavernous A-V anastomoses are described as being in the peripheral part of the cavernous body, thus providing the shortest way of shunting blood. In our own experience, it has not been possible to demonstrate a venous system inside the cavernous bodies. This has also been the experience of Goldstein and Fitzpatrick (1980).

In 1900, von Ebner described the occurrence of pads protruding into arteries with a lumen of 0.2–1.0 mm (Figure 8). These structures have since been found in almost all parts of the arterial tree supplying the erectile tissue as far back as the penile artery after it passes the urogenital diaphragm (Rotter and Schürmann, 1950) (although denied by a single researcher—Deysach, 1939). The pads are characterized by longitudinally oriented smooth-muscle cells surrounded by a splitting of the internal elastic membrane of the arterial wall (Figure 8). A pad may be seen almost completely blocking the lumen over a distance of 1–3 mm. A detailed study of these pads was performed by Kiss (1921).

From anatomical studies the pads have had attributed to them the regulatory

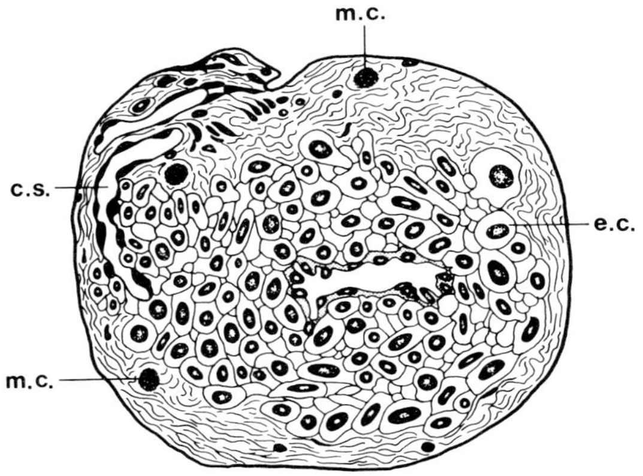

Figure 7. Schematic drawing of an intracavernous helicine artery (diameter 0.08 mm) cut at the opening site into the cavernous tissue. The light cells (e.c.) are epithelioid cells, characteristic of the arteriovenous shunts; m.c. are scattered mast cells, often found in the cavernous tissue; and c.s. is cavernous space lined with endothelial cells.

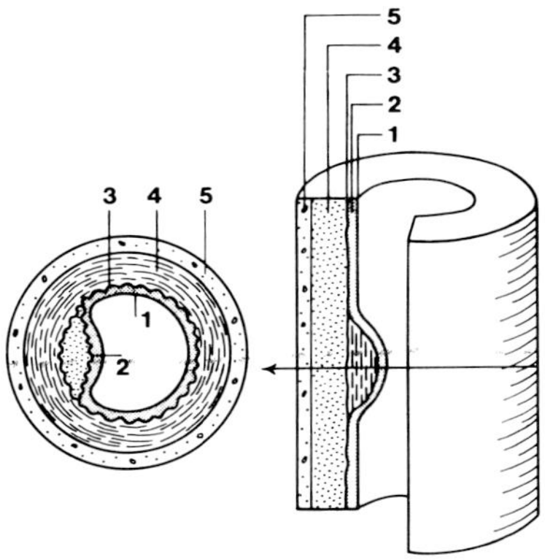

Figure 8. Schematic drawing of the penile artery with an Ebner pad (cushion) protruding into the lumen. (1) Endothelial lining with (2) subendothelial layer, both covering the pad, which consists of longitudinally oriented smooth-muscle cells, active when the penis is flaccid. The tunica elastica (3) splits up and surrounds the pad. (4) The medial layer of the wall with circular smooth-muscle orientation. (5) The loose adventital layer.

mechanism of flaccidity and erection, as well as being a specific site of pathological degenerative changes (Rotter and Schürmann, 1950; Ružbarský and Michal, 1977). (For a discussion of pathology, see Chapter 5.) The pads—when contracted—protrude maximally into the lumen and thereby provide an effective resistance system. By relaxation, the lumen increases, thereby facilitating fluid passage. A serious attack on the normality of these pads has been made recently by Newman and Tchertkoff (1980). They claim, on the basis of the dissection of five adults (18–58 years old) and one stillborn, that the cushions that they identified in arteries as well as in veins in the adult cadavers are nonfunctional structures that develop during the aging process or possibly as a pathological phenomenon.

The venous drainage mainly takes place through the systems of the deep central vein and the deep dorsal vein. Blood in the central area of the cavernous bodies is supposed to be drained into the deep vein through short postcavernous veins collecting blood from the interstices and from the capillaries in the intracavernous tissue. Direct passage has been postulated on the basis of observation of "sluice valves" in deep veins in mammals not possessing an os penis (Deysach, 1939). The thin-walled deep veins leave the cavernous bodies in the area where the bodies diverge and drain to the prostatic venous plexus.

The deep dorsal vein, which in some areas can be seen as a single vessel (Figure 4) or as a richly anastomosizing net (Figure 6), receives its blood from the convolute veins of the glans, via the circumflex veins from the spongiose body and via the venae emissariae from the cavernous bodies. These are thin-walled passages through the tunica albuginea that collect blood mainly from the peripheral part of the erectile tissue. Valves with smooth-muscle content have been found in these communications by Fitzpatrick (1980). Communications to the subcutaneous dorsal vein exist. In this way, the subcutis and the skin may drain through the deep dorsal vein, which via the arcuate veins under the pelvic arch continues into the vesicoprostatic venous plexus and communicates with the vessels from the deep veins.

The deep dorsal vein and its contributions on the dorsum of the penis are extremely thick-walled. This vein also contains valves but rather of the type seen in the veins of the lower extremities (Fitzpatrick, 1975). The main structure is the muscular longitudinal layer, but circular muscular layers exist as well as a very well-pronounced intimal layer bulging into the lumen.

Anatomists have several times, on the basis of their structural descriptions, tried to advance a theory of the mechanism of erection. For a detailed overview, see Kiss (1921). The most widely accepted theory is the one formulated by Conti (1952). With some modifications, it is depicted schematically in Figures 9 and 10.

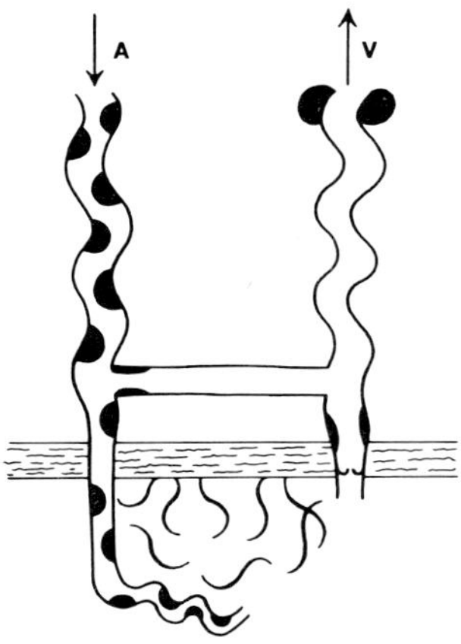

Figure 9. A schematic presentation of the hypothesized direction of blood flow in the flaccid state. A is the tortuous arterial inflow with contracted and protruding pads in the lumen. The blood is supposed to be shunted via the open canal (A-V shunt) into the wide-open vein and to leave through this vein. At the venous outlet (V), a circular sphincter placed under the pelvic arch is relaxed in this state. A modest amount of blood runs through the tunica albuginea into the cavernous space and the capillary system of the cavernous tissue. The drainage is via the open vein, which is provided with valves preventing flow (cf. Figure 10).

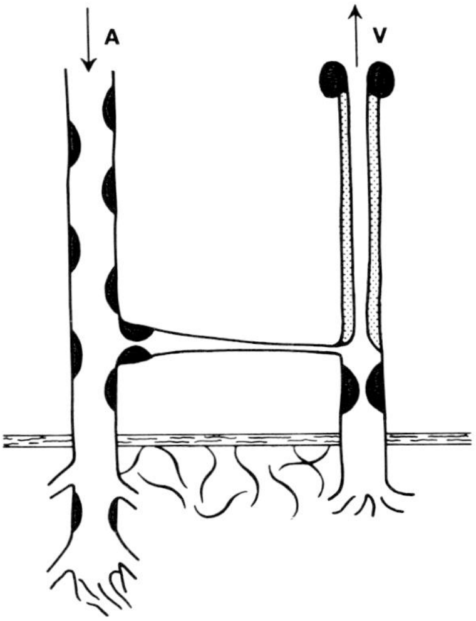

Figure 10. Schematic drawing of circulatory conditions in the erect penis (cf. Figure 9 for flaccid state). The blood flows into the artery (A), now stretched out and with relaxed and flattened Ebner pads in the lumen. The A-V shunt is closed, and the flow of blood continues into the now expanding cavernous space. The return of blood is hampered by closure of the outlet veins, partly by contracted luminal pads and partly by constriction of the wall. The sphincter at the top may also prevent blood from escaping.

In the flaccid state, the arterial cushions are contracted and the course of the artery is tortuous. The arteriovenous shunts are open and the venous drainage free. A circular sphincter (Figures 9 and 10) just under the pelvic arch has recently been described (Haines, 1970). This is supposed to be open in the flaccid state. A modest amount of blood is supposed to pour into the erectile tissue for nutritive purposes, running partly through the helicine arteries and partly into the capillaries of the smooth muscle framework. Through the veins (where valves are present), the blood leaves via the tortuous dorsal venous system or through the deep veins.

In the erect state, the vessels stretch out and the arterial smooth-muscle cushions relax, the arteriovenous shunts close, and free passage of arterial blood is established. This permits the pressure head of the arterial system present in the cavernous spaces to fill with blood, thereby stretching the tunica albuginea. This will passively close off the deep venous drainage, which does not have a structural frame to prevent it from collapsing inside the now formed high-pressure chamber. The outflow of the tunica albuginea, on the other hand, would not be hindered, as the thin-walled veins piercing this structure would expand by the stretching of the tunica. On the outside of the tunica, muscular pads or the muscular walls of the contributions to the deep dorsal vein prevent the escape of blood from the erect organ, possibly in concert with closure in the valve system. Further, the presence of a sphincter centrally around the arcuate vein prevents loss of blood from the erect penis and even allows for regulation during erection.

It must be realized that this theory is based on anatomical studies and not, as shall be described later, on experimental or functional studies.

The Nerve Supply

Erection may be provoked from the brain (psychogenic erection) or from spinal centers (reflexogenic erection). Autonomic and somatic nerves supply the penis (Figure 11). A description of the nerves to the penis was given by Eckhard (1869), who also demonstrated that electrical stimulation of the nerves from the sacral roots produced erection in the dog. It was later found that stimulation of the hypogastric nerve was also able to produce erection. This was also demonstrated in the rabbit by Eckhard (1869) but was not replicated in the dog. Anatomically, the pelvic nerves—nervi erigentes—together with the hypogastric plexus form the prostatic and cavernous plexuses. The sympathetic contributions to these arise as postganglionic as well as preganglionic fibers from the inferior mesenteric ganglion of the abdomen and reach the ganglion at the cord level T12–L1 and L2. The hypogastric plexus crosses the pelvic brim in close association with blood vessels. They flank the rectum and the adjacent parts of the bladder and the seminal vesicles. Also supplying the plexus are the pelvic splanchnic

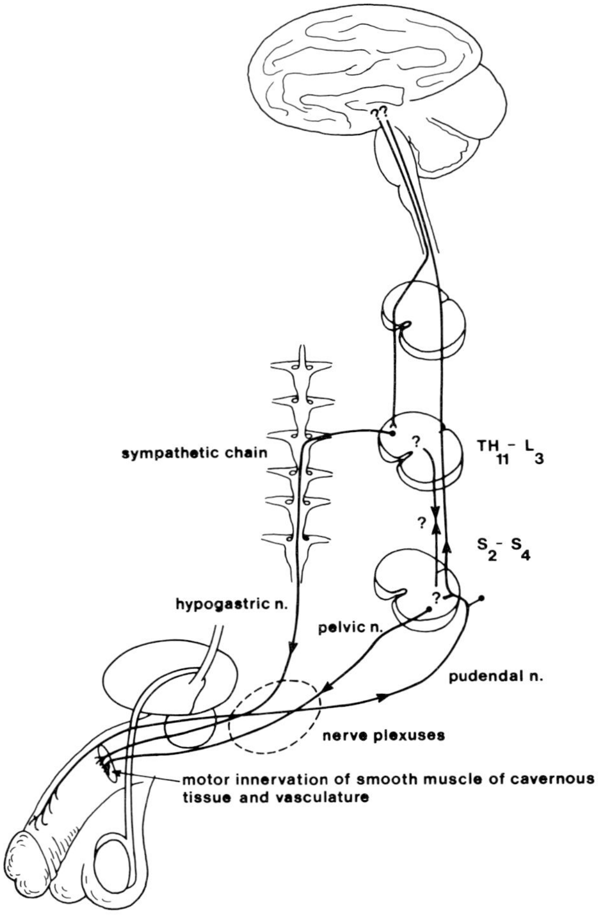

Figure 11. Schematic presentation of the nervous system involved in penile erection. Innervation of the penis is from three sources: somatic, sympathetic, and parasympathetic. Somatic sensory fibers run in the pudendal nerve while the motor innervation of the smooth muscles of the vessels and of the tissue of the cavernous bodies derives from the hypogastric nerve and the pelvic nerves (nervi erigentes) forming the nerve plexuses of the pelvis. Besides the innervation shown, other male genital organs receive fibers from the sympathetic and the parasympathetic systems. The question marks indicate the uncertainty of the synaptic transmissions and connections between a sacral and a lumbar center as well as the cerebral connections in the human.

nerves or the nervi erigentes (the sacral parasympathetic) from the second, third, and fourth sacral nerves. From the inferior hypogastric plexus, which carries sympathetic as well as parasympathetic elements, nerves distribute to the prostatic plexus. This plexus is large and extends from the anterior inferior part of the hypogastric plexus lying beside the prostate and gives off branches to the urethra and the seminal vesicles. The most anterior part of the plexus gives rise to the cavernous plexus, which extends to the erectile tissue of the penis. The sympathetic as well as the parasympathetic nerves are distributed to the cavernous body, the glans, and the spongiose body. Both types of nerve comprise the motor component of the erect and the flaccid states of the penis.

The pudendal nerve, which is the somatic, sensory nerve of the penis, is carried through the roots of the second and third sacral segments. It passes downward as a single structure and runs with the pudendal artery into the pudendal canal and forward. After having given off branches to the perineal area, it passes forward as the dorsal nerve of the penis close to the side of the inferior pubic ramus lying superior to the crus and inferior to the urethral sphincter. It gives off branches to the erectile tissue and continues its course at the lateral side of the dorsal artery. It branches off and distributes nerves to the distal two-thirds and also branches around the sides of the organ to reach the undersurface. The cavernous plexus of the penis contains some small ganglia. Neural receptors are found abundantly in the penis. Free nerve endings are found in the epithelium of the glans, the prepuce, and the mucosa, as well as in the connective tissue of the skin and the urethra. Besides the Meissner's corpuscles, other types of end bulbs, as well as Pacinian corpuscles are located along the dorsal vein of the penis, especially in the deep layers of the connective tissue of the glans and under the covering of the cavernous bodies.

Development of the External Genitalia

During the second month in the embryonic state, at a time when the urogenital sinus has been divided, an elevation arises from the urogenital diaphragm

Table I. Homologous Structures in Male and Female External Genitalia

♂	♀
Glans penis	Glans clitoridis
Urethral surface of penis	Labia minora
Cavernous bodies of penis	Cavernous bodies of clitoris
Spongiose body of penis	Vestibular bulb
Scrotum	Labia majora
Scrotal raphe	Posterior commissure

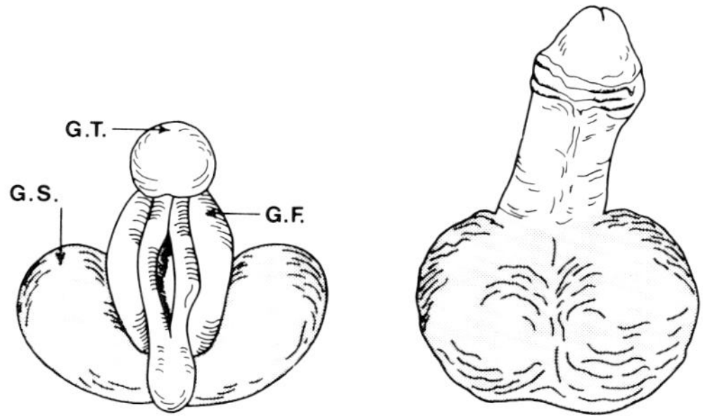

Figure 12. Schematic drawing of the development of the male external genitalia. G.T. = genital tubercle. G.F. = genital fold. G.S. = genital swelling. For explanation see text.

called the *genital tubercle*. Below the tubercle, a groove appears flanked by two ridges—the genital folds. A further pair of prominent folds appears somewhat later. These are the genital swellings (labioscrotal folds) lateral to the genital folds.

The differentiation in the male now starts with elongation of the genital folds producing a penis. The groove that begins to roll in as a urethral canal forms the urethra. Closure of this groove is completed at about the third month. The genital swellings migrate caudally to the base of the penis, where they fuse in the midline to form the scrotum. Figure 12 demonstrates this development. In Table I, the homologous structures of the male and the female genitalia are depicted. The growth of the penis in late human fetal life and during childhood up to adulthood is shown in Figure 13.

It has been known for a long time that the internal secretion of androgens in the male fetus is responsible for the development of the external male genitalia. The experimental evidence was the observation that intrauterine castration of a

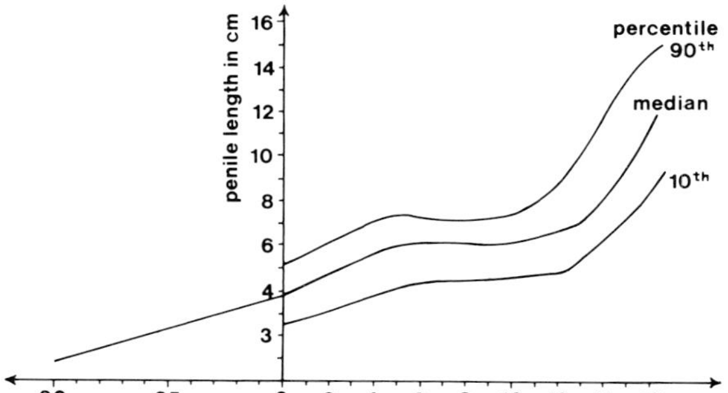

Figure 13. Values for length of penis *in utero*, during childhood, and during adolescence. (Modified after Smith, 1977.)

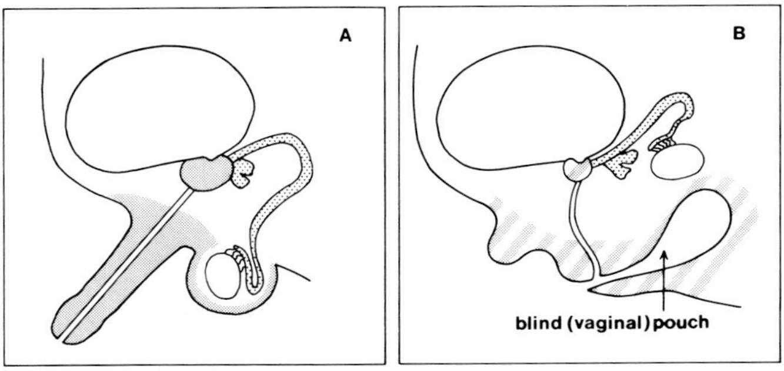

Figure 14. Schematic demonstration of external male genitalia in normal development (A) and in pseudohermaphroditism (B). The solid hatched area indicates the dihydrotestosterone-dependent area in normal development, and the striped hatched area indicates the dihydrotestosterone-dependent area where this influence has not taken place. (Modified after Imperato-McGinley and Peterson, 1976.)

male fetus abolishes the normal development of external genitalia (Jost, 1953). It was later shown that in the human fetus, the endocrine function of the testis, with production and release of testosterone, accelerates at the eighth fetal week and subsides 16 to 20 weeks later (Winter *et al.*, 1977).

The recent description of a group of male pseudohermaphrodites (Imperato-McGinley *et al.*, 1974, 1979) has, however, brought doubt about the role of testosterone as the peripherally acting hormone in normal male development. These men do not have the enzyme 5α reductase that converts testosterone to dihydrotestosterone, a process normally taking place in the peripheral tissue. At birth, the visible defect is limited to the external genitalia: the testes present as inguinal or labial masses, and there are a labia-like scrotum, a urogenital sinus (vaginal pouch), and a clitoral-like phallus (Figure 14). The boys are often reared as "girls," but when the age of puberty is reached, a dramatic change is observed. The phallus enlarges and becomes a functional penis, sperm production is initiated, and the voice deepens. Several of the observed cases have changed from their feminine role to a male pattern with heterosexual interest in females.

The observation of this malfunction has led to the recognition of dihydrotestosterone as the androgen necessary for the intrauterine differentiation to a phenotypic male, while testosterone at puberty appears responsible for the secondary development into the anatomical and functional state of an adult male.

Conclusion

Thus, while more is being learned regarding the anatomical structure of the penis, the complete picture concerning the vascular architecture and its connection with the nervous system has yet to be established. New techniques in the study of penile anatomy are required.

References

Clara, M. (1956). *Anatomie der arterio-venose Anastomosen*. Wien: Springer Verlag.

Conti, G. (1952). L'erection du penis human et ses basis morphologicovasculaires. *Acta Anatomica, 14*, 217–262.

Conti, G. (1953). Über das Vorkommen von Sperrvorrichtungen in Arterien mit spezieller Berucksichtigung der "gestielten Polster." *Acta Anatomica, 18*, 234–255.

Deysach, L. J. (1939). The comparative morphology of the erectile tissue of the penis with especial emphasis on the probable mechanism of erection. *American Journal of Anatomy, 64*, 111–131.

Ebner, V. von (1900). Über klappenartige Vorrichtungen in der Arterien der Schwellkorper. *Anatomische Anzeige, 18*, 79–81.

Eckhard, C. (1869). *Beitrage zur Anatomie und Physiologie*, Vol. 4, pp. 69–88. Giessen: Emil Roth Verlag.

Fitzpatrick, T. J. (1975). A cavernosogram study of the valvular competence of the human deep dorsal vein. *Journal of Urology, 113*, 497–500.

Fitzpatrick, T. J. (1980). Presented at the *Second International Conference on Vasculogenic Impotence*, Monaco, Oct. 8–12.

Forster, A. (1903). Beitrage zur Anatomie der ausseren mannlichen Geschlechtsorgane des Menschen. *Zeitschrift für Morphologie und Antropologie, 6*, 435–501.

Gebhard, P. H., and Johnson, A. B. (1979). *The Kinsey Data: Marginal Tabulation of the 1938–1963 Interviews Conducted by the Institute for Sex Research*. Philadelphia: W. B. Saunders.

Goldstein, A. N. B., and Fitzpatrick, T. J. (1980). Presented at the *Second International Conference on Vasculogenic Impotence*, Monaco, Oct. 8–12.

Haines, R. W. (1970). An unstriped sphincter of the dorsal vein of the penis. *Journal of Anatomy, 107*, 385–386.

Imperato-McGinley, J., and Peterson, R. E. (1976). Male pseudohermaphroditism: The complexities of male phenotypic development. *The American Journal of Medicine, 61*, 251–272.

Imperato-McGinley, J., Guerrero, L., Gautier, T., and Peterson, R. E. (1974). Steroid 5α-reductase deficiency in man: An inherited form of male pseudohermaphroditism. *Science, 186*, 1213–1215.

Imperato-McGinley, J., Petersen, R. E., Gautier, T., and Sturla, E. (1979). Male pseudohermaphroditism secondary to 5α-reductase deficiency—a model for the role of androgens in both the development of the male phenotype and the evolution of a male gender identity. *Journal of Steroid Biochemistry, 11*, 643–645.

Jost, A. (1953). Problems of fetal endocrinology: The gonadal and hypophyseal hormones. *Recent Progress in Hormone Research, 8*, 379–418.

Kiss, F. (1921). Anatomisch-histologische Untersuchungen uber die Erecktion. *Zeitschrift für Anatomie und Entwicklungsgeschichte, 61*, 455–521.

Langer, C. (1862). Über das Gefassystem der mannlichen Schwell-organe. *Sitzungsbericht der Wiener Akademie, 46*, 120–169.

Loeb, H. (1899). Harnrohrenkapacitat und Tripperspritzen. *Munchener Medicinische Wochenschrift, 46*, 1016–1019.

Marberger, H. (1974). The mechanisms of ejaculation. In E. Coutinho and F. Fuchs (Eds.), *Physiology and Genetics of Reproduction*. New York: Plenum.

Masters, W. H., and Johnson, V. E. (1966). *Human Sexual Response*. Boston: Little, Brown.

Müller, J. (1840). *Handbuch der Physiologie des Menschen*. Stuttgart.
Newman, H. F., and Tchertkoff, V. (1980). Penile vascular cushions and erection. *Investigative Urology*, *18*, 43–45.
Newman, H. F., Northup, J. D., and Devlin, J. (1964). Mechanism of human penile erection. *Investigative Urology*, *1*, 350–353.
Piesol, G. A. (1907). *Human Anatomy*. Philadelphia: Lippincott.
Rotter, W., and Schürmann, R. (1950). Die Blutgefasse des menschlichen Penis. Beitrag zur Orthologie und Pathologie der Regulationssysteme des peripheren Kreislaufs (arterio-venose Anastomosen, Sperrarterien und Drosselvenen). *Virchows Archiv*, *318*, 352–393.
Ružbarský, V., and Michal, V. (1977). Morphologic changes in the arterial bed of the penis with aging. *Investigative Urology*, *15*, 194–199.
Smith, D. W. (1977). Micropenis and its management. In R. J. Blandau and D. Bergsma (Eds.), *Morphogenesis and Malformation of the Genital System*. New York: Alan R. Liss.
Stieve, H. (1930). In V. Mollendorph (Ed.), *Handbuch der Gewebelehre des Menschen*, Vol. 7. Berlin: Springer Verlag.
Wagner, G. (1976). *Physiological Responses of the Sexually Stimulated Male in the Laboratory*. 16 mm colour film, Copenhagen/New York.
Watzka, M. (1936). Über Gefasssperren, arteriovenose Anastomosen und den Erythrocytenabbau im Rinderlymphknoten. *Zeitschrift für Mikroskopisch-Anatomische Forschung*, *39*, 250–262.
Winter, J. S. D., Faiman, C., and Reyes, F. I. (1977). Sex steroid production by the human fetus: Its role in morphogenesis and control by gonadotropins. In R. J. Blandau and D. Bergsma (Eds.), *Morphogenesis and Malformation of the Genital System*. New York: Allan R. Liss.

CHAPTER 2

Erection

Physiology and Endocrinology

GORM WAGNER

Penile erection can be defined as a state in which the penis increases in volume and in the standing young man finally presents with an angle between 0 and 45 degrees from the horizontal. In this state, the penis feels rigid in the shaft, and the glans gives under moderate pressure between two fingers. The phenomenon is based on the development of an intracavernous pressure close to the mean arterial pressure. The angling depends on the size of and the pressure in the organ. Through adulthood, the angling normally decreases, perhaps because of a decrease in the maintenance pressure and/or because of a gradual slackening of the suspensory ligaments.

Figure 15 shows the self-measured length and circumference of the flaccid and erect penis in a large group of American white men (Gebhard and Johnson, 1979). It can be seen that in this group there is a considerable range of values. Unfortunately, from these figures, it is not possible to tell the increase in volume in individuals. This information could be of clinical value in cases where a man is concerned about the size of his penis. A very wide range is obtained when volume increase is calculated from these data. The major part of the experimental population exhibits a volume increase with a range from 60 to 150 ml from the flaccid to the erect state.

In a more objective study, Shirai *et al.* (1976) studied the accumulation of blood in the penis during erection by radioisotope penography, making use of the subjects' own red blood cells labeled with 99m Tc. They found a mean increase of 8 times in the intrapenile blood volume from flaccidity to erection, with a range from 4 to 11 times in six cases of full erection. If these figures are used in comparison with the calculated volume (62 ml) from objective measures (p. 7, Chapter 1), and it is assumed that the increase in volume of the penis is 100%, the average

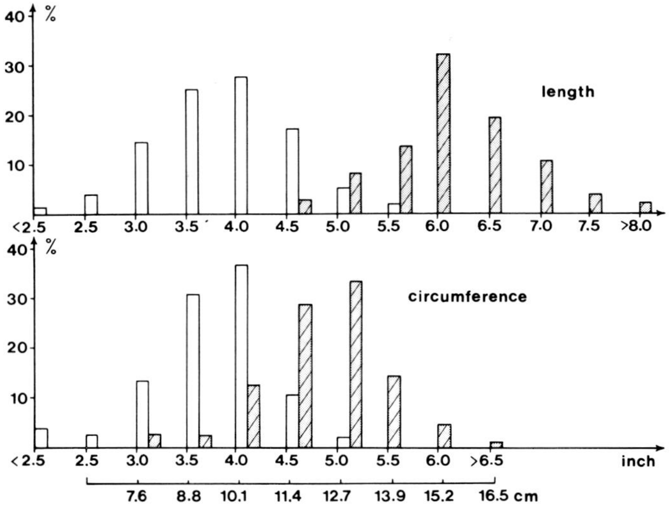

Figure 15. Length and circumference of the penis in the state of flaccidity (white columns) and erection (hatched columns). The material comprises self-measured figures in 2,310 white American males. Tabulated to nearest half inch after the Kinsey data, as reported by Gebhard and Johnson (1979). (The volume increase is due equally to increase in length and increase in circumference.)

blood increase of eightfold would mean that the average blood content of the flaccid penis would be about 8 ml.

The first sign of tumescence is an increase in length slightly before the increase in circumference. At sufficiently intense stimulation, the volume increases first slowly and then more rapidly. The cycle of penile erection can be divided into four phases (see Table II). From Figure 16, it can be seen that full erection is not obtained until somewhat later than full tumescence.

This full tumescence prior to the buildup of intracavernous pressure necessary to lift the penis into erection was recently studied by Metz and Wagner (unpublished). In six male cadavers, the cavernous bodies were cannulated at one side for saline infusion by a constant infusion pump and on the other side for measurement of intracavernous pressure. A strain gauge around the penis measured circumferential changes. The infusion was increased in stepwise fashion in order to obtain an erection judged by the lifting of the penis from the supporting thigh. Although the maximal circumference was obtained, the erection did not occur until after the intracavernous pressure had increased further. In these cases, the organ lifted at a pressure from 85 to 105 mm Hg. The infusion rate necessary to obtain rigidity and erection varied from 45 to 65 ml/min, but once the erection was established, a perfusion of 30–50 ml/min was sufficient to maintain this state.

Table II. The Four Phases of the Erectile Cycle (cf. Figures 16 and 17)

I.	*Resting phase*: constant volume, intracavernous pressure, and blood flow rate.
II.	*Tumescence phase*: volume increases, and there is a slight increase in intracavernous pressure. The duration of this phase is age-dependent and is influenced by the strength and the reception of the sexual stimulation.
III.	*Erection phase*: volume is constant, and the intracavernous pressure has increased to at least 80 mm Hg.
IVa.	*Detumescence phase (rapid)*: stiffness is lost and volume decreases.
IVb.	*Detumescence phase (slow), or restitution phase*: volume returns to basal value.

These flows are of the same order of magnitude necessary to provide artificial erection in a fully anesthetized man (cf. p. 124, Chapter 8). This finding supports the necessity of finding whether a given tumescence is identical with stiffness when nocturnal penile tumescence is investigated in a case of erectile dysfunction (cf. p. 104, Chapter 8).

The outflow, which in a steady state (i.e., constant volume) equals inflow, expresses the blood flow rate of the tissue. The xenon washout technique (described in Chapter 8) has indicated a flow rate of 2.5–8 ml in the flaccid state (Wagner and Uhrenholdt, 1978). Ishii (1978) found slightly lower values, although he used an assumption in the calculation that gave higher results. The λ value in our experiments is set at 0.7 (the blood-to-tissue partition coefficient), while in Phases II and III of erection, the λ is 0.85 because of the increase in blood volume of the cavernous spaces. The use of different λ values does not result in major differences, as the changes in outflow from flaccid to erect and from erect to flaccid are significant (Figure 17). The characteristic finding of a reduced or maintained outflow during tumescence suggests an active regulation of the outlet.

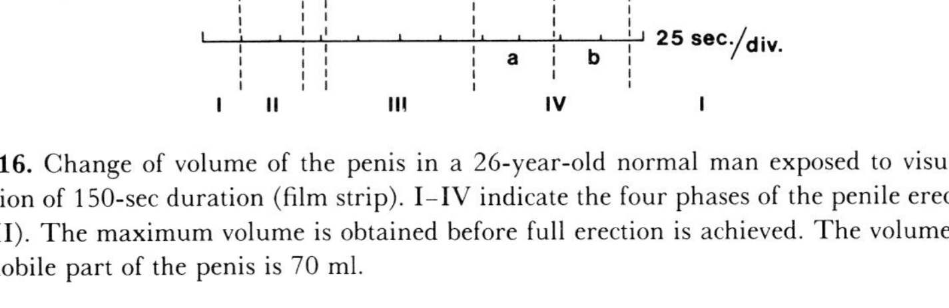

Figure 16. Change of volume of the penis in a 26-year-old normal man exposed to visual sexual stimulation of 150-sec duration (film strip). I–IV indicate the four phases of the penile erectile cycle (Table II). The maximum volume is obtained before full erection is achieved. The volume increase of the mobile part of the penis is 70 ml.

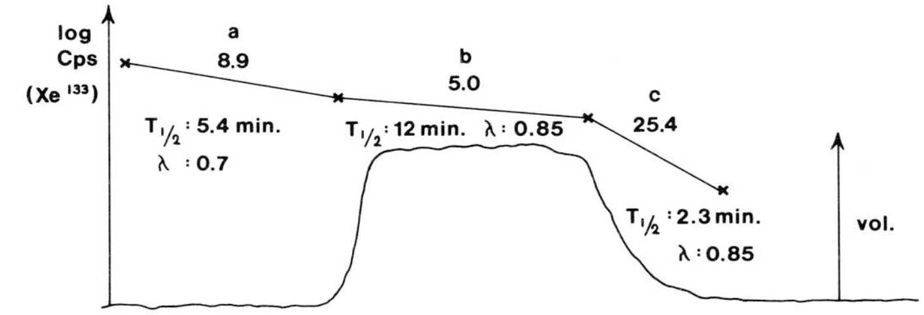

Figure 17. The washout of radioactive xenon (Xe^{133}) from an intracavernous deposit during period of flaccidity (a), tumescence and erection (b), and detumescence (c). The λ-value is changed when the volume of blood in the corpus cavernosum increases. Ordinate: log value of measured radioactive values from an experiment. It is seen that some reduction in calculated flow (8.9–5.0 ml/min/100 g) occurs during the tumescence phase. During detumescence (c), the outflow increases to 25.4 ml/min/100 g.

Figure 18 summarizes the simultaneous changes of volume, intracavernous pressure, and outflow from the cavernous bodies during the four phases of a complete erectile cycle. If the outlet is added, the rate of volume increase (ml/min) indicates the arterial flow rate during tumescence. In a young man, as demonstrated in Figure 16, the average arterial influx is (for the whole organ) 90 ml/min. During

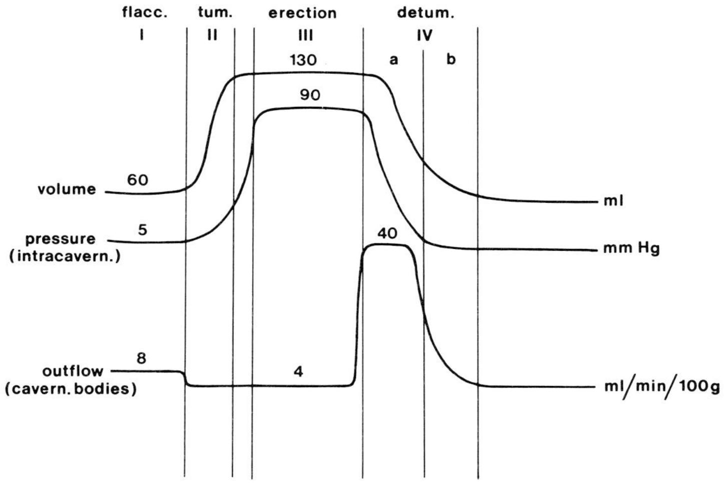

Figure 18. Theoretical presentation of circulatory changes in each of four phases of the penile erectile cycle. Volume of the penis, intracavernous pressure, and outflow from cavernous bodies are depicted with average values and are presented to demonstrate their interrelationship. It should be noted that an intermediate phase exists after the maximum volume has occurred (II) and the maximum pressure is developed (III). During this period, the pressure is built up to that necessary to create rigidity of the cavernous bodies.

the period of 10 sec when the greatest volume increase takes place, the arterial influx equals about 270 ml/min.

In normal young men, the increase in influx from the flaccid phase to the most rapid period of the tumescence phase has been found to be 25-fold to 60-fold. The massive flow increase must require a well coordinated neuromuscular system and a highly expansive arterial bed supplying the cavernous tissue. That Phase II (tumescence) is the one prolonged during aging seems understandable simply from the gradual aging of the arterial system with a slight decrease in distensibility. However, the degree of such changes and their relationship to erectile ability remains to be determined.

The detumescence phase is slower than the tumescence phase (see Figure 16). The drainage time, which is characterized by an initial period with high outflow (up to 50 ml/min), is followed by a period of slow outflow that gradually approaches basal values. It could be argued that the initial drainage is caused by the high intracavernous pressure as the maximum value of 50 ml/min is equivalent to the capacity of the venous drainage system. It fits well with the maintenance flow during artificial erection in the fully anesthetized man or in a cadaver. The slow part of detumescence (Phase IVb) might be caused by contraction of the smooth muscle of the cavernous tissue. Man does not have well-defined retractor muscles like most animals, and the retraction that can be demonstrated experimentally by cold exposure or by sudden distraction is obviously an active process occurring with a speed that resembles smooth-muscle activity.

Table III gives an overview of the smooth-muscle structures that are most likely involved in the erectile cycle and their state of activity during the four phases. During these phases, the glans and the spongiose body do not achieve a pressure increase of the same magnitude as that of the cavernous bodies. No measurements of this pressure increase or of the volume increase that occurs have been reported. Only a few blood flow studies have been performed experimentally with the xenon washout technique. The flow at rest was found to be higher in the glans (15–20 ml/min/100 g tissue) than in the cavernous bodies. At sexual stimulation,

Table III. Phases of Penile Erection Cycle[a]

		I Flaccidity	II Tumescence	III Erection	IVa,b Detumescence
Smooth muscle of	Arterial pads	Contracted	Relaxed	Relaxed	Contracted
	Av shunts	Relaxed	Contracted	Contracted	Relaxed
	Cavernous tissue ("retractor")	Contracted	Relaxed	Relaxed	Contracted
	Venous pads and walls	Relaxed	Contracted	Contracted	Relaxed

[a]The table shows which of the four smooth-muscle sites in the penile circulatory system may be active in the four phases of the penile erectile cycle.

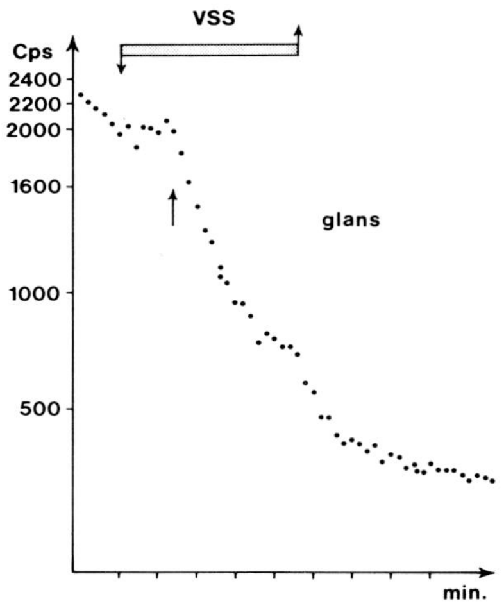

Figure 19. Plotting of washout of radioactive xenon-deposit placed in the glans. The calculated value at rest is 18.2 ml/min/100 g, followed by an almost complete stop in washout when visual sexual stimulation (VSS) is initiated. At the arrow, a sudden increase in outflow occurs. This increase is concomitant with the start of the tumescence phase of the corpus cavernosum. The flow acceleration is calculated to 92 ml/min/100 g and is followed by a slower phase at the end of stimulation and a further decrease in the poststimulatory period.

a slight decrease in flow is seen (possibly concomitant with an increase of volume in the glans). This decrease is followed by a sharp increase in flow at the same time as the increase of volume in the cavernous bodies begins (Figure 19). The calculated flow in the glans during this period is in the range of 80–100ml/min/100 g. The changes in flow could be explained by an initial, slight venous constriction, followed by an increased arterial input, which increases the intraspongiose pressure so as to overcome the venous restriction of flow. Also, a decreased filling of the venous system, occurring when the outflow from the cavernous bodies is diminished, might facilitate an increase of outflow from the glans. The above should be considered a speculative explanation, as too few experiments have been conducted.

Mechanism of Erection

On the basis of anatomical descriptions and functional studies, the theory of the mechanism of erection can be proposed through the following six steps:

1. *Relaxation of Ebner pads (active)*, causing a decrease in resistance to arterial pressure and flow rate.
2. *Dilatation of arterial vasculature (passive and/or active)*, increasing volume and facilitating (a) the arterial pressure head to reach intracavernous spaces and (b) the increase in flow rate.
3. *Closure of A-V (arteriovenous) shunts (active)*, preventing draining from the arterial system.

4. *Relaxation of the smooth muscle of the cavernous tissue (active)*, decreasing the resistance to a volume increase of the cavernous bodies, resulting from the increased arterial flow rate.
5. *Closure (or regulation) of venous bleed valves (active)*, to prevent increased blood volume under developing pressure from escaping.
6. *Stretching of vessels (passive)*, facilitating flow and pressure.

The above processes change the intracavernous space from a low-volume, low-pressure system into the large-volume, high-pressure system needed for the penis to penetrate a slitlike, soft, expandable canal. The low-pressured but enlarged glans may act as a functional cushion, preventing pain or damage in the receiving system. Also, the pressure of the tissue surrounding the outlet of the ejaculatory canal should not exceed that of the high-pressure chamber formed in the bulbar part of the urethra preceding ejaculation.

Discussion of an active venous regulation in Phases II and III of the erectile cycle has been present in the literature for a long time. From present-day findings, it seems clear that an active regulation has to exist because of the following:

1. The measurement of a decreased or maintained flow during tumescence in spite of the large capacity of the drainage system (xenon studies).
2. The observation of diminished outlet of contrast medium from cavernous bodies in Phase II (cf. infusion cavernosography, p. 114).
3. The equivalence of outflow (ml/min) during detumescence in normal erection (plethysmography and xenon studies) with the maintenance flow during artificial erection (during anesthesia).
4. The unexplainable detumescence phase were venous closure passive; that is, closure is due solely to an increase of intracavernous pressure.
5. The impossibility of erection if a fistula has been produced from the cavernous to the spongiose bodies (to bring an end to priapism) and is still open.
6. The description of leakages from the cavernous system leading to erectile dysfunction and the occurrence of erectile ability after surgical closure of the leakages.

Neural Regulation of Erection

A recent electron-microscopic study (McConnell, 1979) of the human corpus cavernosum described the finding of irregularly shaped vesicles of 800–1200 Å in diameter. This type of vesicle found in other tissues has been shown to be peptidergic. Also found were vesicles that could be described as cholinergic and adrenergic. This new description makes it no clearer which neuromuscular transmission system is involved in erection. A further complication is that some smooth-muscle groups (in the Ebner pads and the cavernous tissue) stay active in order to keep the penis flaccid. Thus, these muscles have to relax while the muscle groups in the A-V shunts and those of the drainage system have to contract in order to shift from flaccidity to erection.

The nature of the neural regulation has been the subject of a long-standing dispute in the physiological literature. Langley and Anderson (1895), in their classic and comprehensive study of the pelvic nerves, put forward the parasympathetic nerves from the sacral roots as the only pathway for vasodilation. This assumption was maintained by Semans and Langworthy (1938), although other studies showed neural pathways through the sympathetic hypogastric nerve (Eckhard, 1876; Bacq, 1935). The other major issue has been whether the vasodilation is mediated through cholinergic nerves, as proposed by Henderson and Roepke (1933) and Bacq (1935) but later denied by Luduena and Grigas (1966) and Dorr and Brody (1967). In man, erection can be produced by electrical stimulation of the S2, S3, or S4 roots (Habib, 1967), but only two of the roots are effective in any one man (G. S. Brindley, personal communication, 1980). Habib's investigations, done on five paraplegic patients, indicated that S3 was the major erectile root of the two roots in four patients and that S2 was the major root in one man.

While only a few human pharmacological studies exist, extensive physiological studies of the neural regulation of penile function have been carried out in the rabbit (for a survey, see Sjöstrand and Klinge, 1979). Sjöstrand and Klinge have criticized earlier investigations on the basis of technical errors. Their main finding in the rabbit is the demonstration of two sets of vasodilator fibers, both with pelvic ganglionic relays. One set is the pelvic parasympathetic nerves, mainly with noncholinergic postganglionic neurons, and the other set derives from the sympathetic hypogastric nerves, partly with cholinergic postganglionic neurons, which may work as vasodilators and as suppressors of the adrenergic vasoconstrictor system that derives from the sacrococcygeal part of the sympathetic chain. If the adrenergic vasoconstrictor system is cut, protrusion of the penis occurs, indicating that a constant adrenergic tone is necessary to keep the vasoconstriction working and thereby keeping the penis flaccid. Some time after cutting, autoregulation of penile size is established. No observation of blood flow or of venous regulation of flow was attempted (Sjöstrand and Klinge, 1979).

The complexity of the local neural regulation of the flow pressure in the penis thus makes studies of man difficult to undertake. In recent experiments carried out in the human (Wagner and Brindley, 1978), after atropine infusion to normal, young subjects (0.035 mg/kg) no change in the ability to produce a rapid and full erection was observed, whether the erection was provoked by visual stimulation or by local vibration. Even larger doses of atropine given to baboons could not prevent erection provoked by the electrical stimulation of sacral roots.

In other experiments with adrenergic blocking agents (β-blocker propranolol) in doses of 80 mg/day or the α-blocking agent (phenoxybenzamine) in doses of 40–120 mg daily, it was not possible to impair the speed of erection or the stiffness of the penis. No simultaneous flow studies were conducted. One observation could support the view of an adrenergic vasoconstrictor tone during flaccidity. In the men receiving the α blocking agent, the length of the penis increased in some subjects (about 2 cm).

In summary, these findings do not support the concept of a dominance of either a cholinergic or an adrenergic neurotransmission system in the tumescence or erection phases, but they possibly support the concept of an adrenergic system preventing erection.

Recently, Larsson *et al.* (1977) have demonstrated the presence of vasoactive polypeptide (VIP) in the male genital tract of the cat. Although the demonstration of VIP in the cavernous bodies was of a low level, they postulated the possible role of VIP as a local neurotransmitter. This finding has led us to study the human penis, and preliminary findings indicate a very high concentration of VIP in erectile tissue. The main physiological effect of injected VIP in other genital organs is a short-lasting relaxation of smooth-muscle activity (Ottesen *et al.*, 1979).

Hormones and Erection

Since antiquity, it has been known that a relation exists between the testes and sexual function. In antiquity and until recent times, castration has been performed to lower sexual activity in men. During the seventeenth and eighteenth centuries, boys were castrated in order to preserve their beautiful singing voices.

The development of secondary sex characteristics is dependent on the occurrence of androgen production and secretion, although maintenance of these features does not seem to be hormone-dependent. It is known that boys with low testosterone plasma concentrations are able to erect. It is also known that the castration of adult men, with a consequent drop in circulating hormone concentration, produces varied results. In large series of castrated adults (mainly sex offenders), it can be observed that some lose their sexual interest and activity after a few months, while others keep almost normal sexual activity for up to 10 years. There are few data on the direct effect of androgens on erectile ability. A recent study does, however, shed some light on this relationship (Davidson *et al.*, 1979; also see Chapter 10). It can be speculated that the effect of androgen on erection is quantitative rather than qualitative.

The plasma concentration of testosterone during the male life cycle is shown in Figure 20, where it can be seen that a mean plasma level of around 600 ng/100 ml is retained from the age of 20 to close to 60. From the sixth decade and during the rest of senescence, the concentration falls. The range of values is, how-

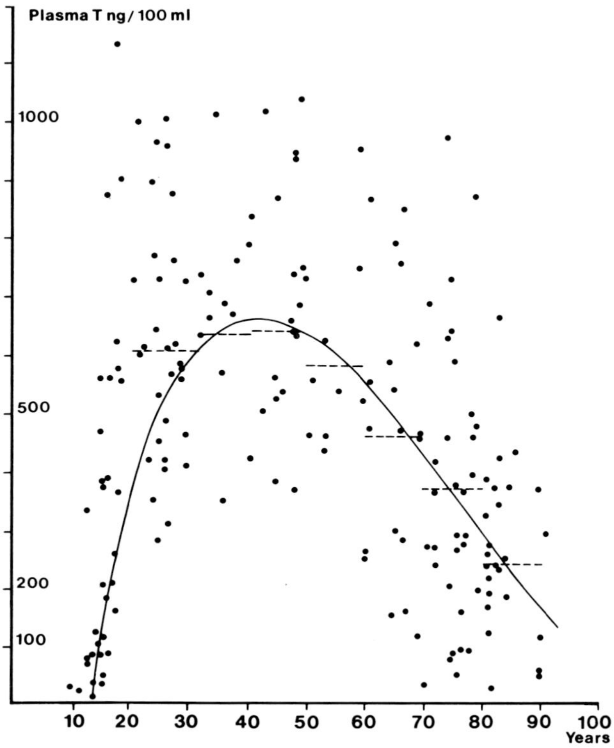

Figure 20. Variation of concentration of plasma testosterone (free and bound) with age in normal men. Dotted lines indicate mean value for each 10-year group. (Modified from Vermeulen *et al.*, 1972.)

ever, very large. It is not known whether any given plasma concentration is the limit for a certain change in sexual activity or in erectile capacity.

Table IV shows variations in the age groups and the simultaneous fall in the percentage of free testosterone with increasing age. This fall is due to increased production of serum-hormone-binding globulin (SHBG). It is a matter of dispute, however, whether the concentration (even of free hormone) is of importance in the qualitative functions of the respondent cells. It could very well be a matter of differential receptivity, which would allow for a wide interpretation of the unclear (and unpredictable) results of intake of androgen in poorly defined groups of "impotent" men.

Also changing concomitantly with age is the frequency of intercourse. In

Table IV. Variation of Testosterone Plasma Concentration, Metabolic Clearance, and Production Rate during Male Adulthood[a]

Age in years	Mean ±SEM	Plasma level (ng/100 ml) range	Free percentage mean ±SEM	Metabolic clearance rate ($1/m^2/24$ h)	Blood production rate (mg/24 h)
20–30	614±43	280–1205			
30–40	634±41	350–1010	2.08±0.8	640±25	6.6±0.5
40–50	640±49	255–1025			
50–60	582±62	255–950	1.68±0.09		
60–70	462±70	120–870			
70–80	373±46	38–850	1.36±0.09	530±35	4.0±0.6
80–90	245±26	28–390			

[a]Modified from Vermeulen *et al.* (1972).

2801 urological patients, as described by Pearlman and Kobashi (1972), 88% who were younger than 20 had intercourse more than once a week, 80% had more than weekly intercourse in the fourth decade, 68% in the fifth, 50% in the sixth, and 25% in the seventh, while 10% continued this activity into the eighth decade.

The secretion of testosterone is not constant, but comes in short spurts, six or seven times a day, with increments preceded some 3 h by a release of luteinizing hormone. The mean concentration shows a clear diurnal variation, with a high concentration in the morning. As both shorter and longer plasma variations occur, it should be understood that a single plasma determination may be misleading. During the night, the concentrations vary and the peak values occur at the time of the REM phases of sleep. Erections during these phases are not necessarily caused by these acute elevations in hormone level. Sexual intercourse has been found to be followed by an elevation in plasma testosterone, while masturbation was not followed by any surge (Fox *et al.*, 1972).

Conclusion

Studies of the mechanisms of human penile erection are few. Definitions of erection and analysis of the complicated neural and circulatory conditions during flaccidity and erection are a basic necessity. These are required for an understanding of normal penile function, which, in turn, is necessary for an understanding of pathophysiology. The missing link is understanding the neurotransmission system. With the necessity of functional diagnostic procedures, the need for basic research is urgent.

References

Bacq, Z. M. (1935). Recherches sur la physiologie et la pharmacologie du système nerveux autonome. *Archives Internationales de Physiologie*, *40*, 311–321.

Davidson, J. M., Camorgo, C. A., and Smith, E. R. (1979). Effects of androgen on sexual behaviour in hypogonadal men. *Journal of Clinical Endocrinology and Metabolism*, *48*, 955–958.

Dorr, L. D., and Brody, M. J. (1967). Hemodynamic mechanisms of erection in the canine penis. *American Journal of Physiology*, *213*, 1526–1531.

Eckhard, C. (1876). Über den Verlauf der nn. erigentes innerhalb des Rückenmarks und Gehirns. *Beitrage zur Anatomie und Physiologie*, VII Band. Giessen.

Fox, C., Ismail, A., Love, D., Kirkham, K., and Loraine, J. (1972). Studies on the relationship between plasma testosterone levels in human sexual activity. *Journal of Endocrinology*, *52*, 51–54.

Gebhard, P. H., and Johnson, A. B. (1979). *The Kinsey Data: Marginal Tabulations of the 1938–1963 Interviews Conducted by the Institute for Sex Research*, Philadelphia: W. B. Saunders.

Habib, H. N. (1967). Experimental and recent contribution in sacral nerve stimulation for voiding in both man and animal. *British Journal of Urology*, *39*, 73–83.

Henderson, V. E., and Roepke, M. H. (1933). On the mechanism of erection. *American Journal of Physiology*, *106*, 441–448.

Ishii, N. (1978). Hemodynamic mechanism of erection in human penis. *Nippon hinyokika gakkai zasshi*, *69*, 870–877.

Langley, J. N., and Andersen, H. K. (1896). The innervation of the pelvic and adjoining viscera. Part VI. *Journal of Physiology*, *20*, 372–406.

Larsson, L. I., Fahrenkrug, J., and Schaffalitzky de Muckadell, O. B. (1977). Occurrence of nerves containing vasoactive intestinal polypeptide immunoreactivity in the male genital tract. *Life Sciences*, *21*, 503–508.

Luduena, F. P., and Grigas, E. O. (1966). Pharmacological study of autonomic innervation of dog retractor penis. *American Journal of Physiology*, *210*, 435–444.

McConnell, J. A. (1979). EM analysis of the adrenergic and possible peptidergic innervation of the human vas deferens and corpus cavernosum. *The Anatomical Record*, *193*, 618.

Ottesen, B., Ulrichsen, H., Wagner, G., and Fahrenkrug, J. (1979). Vasoactive intestinal polypeptide (VIP) inhibits oxytocin induced activity of the rabbit myometrium. *Acta Physiologica Scandinavica*, *107*, 285–287.

Pearlman, C. K., and Kobashi, L. I. (1972). Frequency of intercourse in men. *The Journal of Urology*, *107*, 298–301.

Semans, J. H., and Langworthy, O. R. (1938). Observations on the neurophysiology of sexual function in the male cat. *Journal of Urology*, *40*, 836–846.

Shirai, M., Nakamura, M., Ishii, N., Mitsaukawa, S., and Sawai, Y. (1976). Determination of intrapenial blood volume using ^{99m}Tc-labeled autogenous red blood cells. *Tohoku Journal of Experimental Medicine*, *120*, 377–383.

Sjöstrand, N. O., and Klinge, E. (1979). Principal mechanisms controlling penile retraction and protrusion in rabbits. *Acta Physiologica Scandinavica*, *106*, 199–214.

Vermeulen, A., Rubens, R., and Verdonck, L. (1972). Testosterone secretion and metabolism in male senescense. *Journal of Clinical Endocrinology*, *34*, 730–735.

Wagner, G., and Brindley, G. S. (1978). Effect of atropine on erection. Presented at *First International Conference on Vasculogenic Impotence*, New York.

Wagner, G., and Uhrenholdt, A. (1978). Blood flow measurement by the clearance method in the human corpus cavernosum in the flaccid and erect states. Presented at the *First International Conference on Vasculogenic Impotence*, New York.

CHAPTER 3

General Medical Disorders and Erectile Failure

GORM WAGNER AND RICHARD GREEN

During illness and convalescence, sexual activity drops in most men. The reasons may be the major impact of being sick, anxiety about the immediate future, or other concerns of the patient. The drop in sexual activity may also be a nonspecific symptom of the disease, or it may be a specific symptom in a neurological disease or in diabetes mellitus.

Frequently, diseases not directly affecting the genital area decrease sexual drive, without necessarily causing erectile problems. A true psychogenic erectile dysfunction secondary to chronic disease may also present where concern about self-esteem and the value of life preoccupies the man. And finally, there may be an organic erectile dysfunction due to lesions of nerves or vessels induced by surgery or localized pathology, or resulting from pharmacological agents. It is the task of the physican to separate these factors and through a comprehensive interview to obtain a clear picture of the symptoms. The further diagnostic strategy depends on these data. In this chapter, we concern ourselves with erectile problems only in relation to diseases other than three major groups that are covered in separate chapters: diabetes mellitus, atherosclerosis, and alcoholism.

It is well known that physicians and patients have a communication problem when sexual inadequacy is not the major focus of their relationship. Both the patient and the doctor are products of the same cultural tradition that generally inhibits their speaking about sexual function. It is the task of the professional to initiate discussion. The lack of specific training in sexuality in medical schools until recent years has prevented physicians from feeling at ease in dealing with sexual matters. It is recommended to those who have had no previous training in medical sexology that they attend postgraduate courses that will bring these topics into their professional life so that this area may become part of their patient care. Newer texts to meet this goal are also available (Green, 1979; Kolodny *et al.*, 1979).

Heart Disease

In well-controlled and well-treated chronic heart disease, sexual activity should not present any great risk since the man will know the degree of strain he is able to endure. A specific group, however, is composed of men who have survived a coronary occlusion. Quite often, as soon as the man is out of acute danger and about to leave the intensive-care unit, he speculates about the possibility of a sexual life similar to that of the preinfarction state. It is common clinical experience that patients encounter problems if questions of their sexuality are not taken up before they leave the hospital. Erectile problems usually do not occur in this phase unless patients are treated with antihypertensive or antidepressant drugs. Clinically, it may not be wise to induce anxiety in the patient by telling him that this particular drug may cause erectile problems. The literature contains case histories in which propranolol (the most commonly used β-blocker) has given rise to "impotence," but they are few and it should not necessarily be considered a side effect of the drug. The erectile failure may be due to a lowering of the blood pressure, which may impede the intracavernous pressure necessary for erection. Also, it may be concomitant to a secondary psychogenic erectile dysfunction in patients who are afraid of coitus and the strain on their injured heart. The formation of "heart clubs" in many hospitals may be of help to some patients but may create concerns in others if such groups are not well guided, as pointed out by Friedman (1978).

The rise in systemic blood pressure during coitus varies according to the sexual situation. In a single experiment (Fox *et al.*, 1972), it was noted that a dose of propranolol sufficient to keep a constant blood pressure during coitus did not affect erection, ejaculation, or orgasm in the male, nor did it affect vaginal lubrication or orgasm in the female. As noted elsewhere, α- or β-blockade does not interfere with erection in normotensive men during controlled laboratory studies (Wagner and Brindley, 1978).

Pulse rate and blood pressure in prone and supine coital positions were examined by Nemec *et al.* (1976), who found no difference in the two positions. In a telemetry study, Hellerstein and Friedman (1970) compared 48 postcoronary patients with 43 noninfarcted but coronary-prone men. The mean maximal heart rate during orgasm (peak of heart activity) was 117 beats/min (range 90–144). The mean value during their usual occupational activity was 120. EKG changes and anginal symptoms were comparable in the two situations. Orgasm from masturbation may induce similar changes (Wagner, 1976).

Another group with heart disease that may complain of sexual dysfunction consists of men on long-term digoxin treatment. In one study, 14 men who had been taking digoxin for at least five years were compared with 12 who were not on this drug; the groups were matched for current cardiac status. Of the men on digoxin, 5 complained of lack of sexual desire and erectile failure, and 6 reported lower frequency of sexual outlet, compared with none in the nondigoxin group. The differences might be explainable by changes in hormonal status: for the digoxin group, estradiol was nearly three times higher, testosterone nearly two-thirds lower, and luteinizing hormone (LH) was nearly one-half lower. However, there was no correlation between level of testosterone or estradiol and sexual functioning (Neri *et al.*, 1980).

Thus, secondary erectile dysfunction may occur in postcoronary patients, but it may be avoidable with sufficient preventive medical counseling and an assurance of assistance if any sexual problems should occur. The same applies to a very special group of men who have had heart transplantation. Of the patients reported by Wolpowitz and Barnard (1978), 25% experienced secondary erectile dysfunction with continued desire for sexual activity. No metabolic, hepatic, or renal dysfunctions were found. They were treated with Pasuma® (containing testosterone, vitamin E, yohimbine, strychnine, ephedrine, and caffeine). All patients who completed one month's treatment reported having regained a satisfactory sexual life. The authors suggested that the erectile failure may have been due to the immunosuppressive treatment in connection with transplantation, a theory that contradicts the experience with renal transplantation, where the erectile dysfunction often disappears during the period of immunosuppression.

Chronic Renal Failure

In uremia, a series of metabolic derangements influencing the male reproductive functions occurs before and after hemodialysis. Low circulating levels of testosterone, Leydig cell abnormalities with a decline in spermatozoa maturation, elevated levels of follicle-stimulating hormone (FSH) and LH, an increase in prolactin levels, and secondary hyperparathyroidism may all occur (Massry *et al.*, 1977; Chopp and Mendez, 1978).

It has been well documented that reduced or partial erectile ability exists in 38–80% of dialysis patients, while 20–55% are completely impotent (Levy, 1976; Abram *et al.*, 1975). Often the condition worsens after the initiation of dialysis. Although the presence of sexual dysfunction has been clearly shown, the mechanisms involved are not clear. The usual low testosterone values found may be increased by the administration of human chorionic gonadotropin or chlomiphene. Prolactin elevation may be seen both with and without simultaneous occurrence of gynecomastia. It seems possible that a deficient feedback mechasism between testosterone and luteinizing hormone-releasing factor (LHRF) exists as in some patients a release of LH can be induced by exogenous LHRF. Some investigators hold prolactin responsible for the low testosterone and suggest an antigonadotropic action at the gonadal level (Zarate *et al.*, 1972).

It has also been proposed that prolactin itself is the cause of the erectile dysfunction. However, the study of Hagen *et al.* (1976) argues against this proposal in that only 12 of their 21 patients on dialysis had elevated prolactin levels. These men were divided equally into groups of dysfunctional and functional men. Treatment with bromocriptine, which lowers prolactin, restored a normal sexual function in some patients without concomitant treatment with testosterone (Bommer *et al.* 1979; Spark *et al.* 1980). The role of prolactin in normal and abnormal sexual behavior and genital function remains to be elucidated. After renal transplantation, testosterone and prolactin levels return to normal and the patients usually regain their normal sexual activity.

Transient erectile problems do occur, however, in some patients who have kidney transplantation as the arterial supply is reduced by the ligation of the internal iliac artery, which is used for arterial supply to the new kidney (Figure 5, Chapter 1). Usually the communicants between the penile arteries are sufficient to establish and maintain erection. If, however, a second renal transplantation is undertaken, erectile failure will most likely follow. Recently, it has been reported that while 10% of patients experienced transient erectile failure after the first transplantation, 65% were unable to erect after the second. Half of these regained some degree of erection within eight months. To avoid this complication, the surgical procedure could be changed to an end-to-side anastomosis to the external iliac artery, thus sparing the ligation of the remaining internal iliac artery (Gittes and Waters, 1979).

On the basis of observations by Loew *et al.* (1975), who found secondary hyperparathyroidism with dialysis, Massry *et al.* (1977) have suggested that parathyroid hormone may play a role in the development of erectile failure. Seven dialysis patients were evaluated for sexual activity and hormonal levels. They had elevated levels of plasma parathyroid hormone (PTH) and low testosterone. Four were impotent. They were treated with 1,25-dihydroxy-vitamin D_3 to produce suppression of the parathyroid glandular activity. In four of the seven, PTH levels fell and testosterone levels rose. In two of the dysfunctional men, with hormonal change, sexual activity changed. In two others, the PTH level did not decrease toward normal, and they remained dysfunctional.

The above findings notwithstanding, little is known about the emotional state of the uremic patient in relation to his sexual activity. We are faced with a group of chronically sick patients burdened by the severity of their disease. This fact cannot be ruled out as part of their malfunction. Thus, close contact between doctor and patient is of great importance in this group.

Chronic Lung Disease

In 90 men with chronic bronchitis, asthma, or emphysema, 19% were found to have erectile failure. From a careful psychic and social evaluation, it appeared that the erectile problems were related not to the pathophysiological aspects of the pulmonary disorder even in advanced cases but to the interpersonal problems created by the disease. Information on sexual matters and on the nature of the disease reduced the incidence of sexual problems (Kass *et al.*, 1972).

Surgery

Major surgery in the thorax or the abdomen, as well as local surgery around the reproductive organs, may cause temporary erectile problems. Two common types of surgery frequently result in specific problems for erection: prostatectomy and ileostomy or colostomy.

Prostate Surgery

The effect of prostatectomy on sexuality varies with the procedure performed. Of all the types of prostatectomy, only perineal prostatectomy, which is rarely performed, produced impotence in a large series of patients. Transurethral (TUR) procedures, done in about 95% of patients, should not threaten potency. A study by Zohar *et al.* (1976) noted that whether the man becomes impotent may have more to do with the surgeon's bedside manner than with his surgical technique. In a study of 15 preoperative, potent prostatectomy patients under age 70, 1 of 7 who received a few minutes of explanation about the forthcoming operation on the first day of hospitalization experienced sexual dysfunction. By contrast, 5 of 8 who did not receive an explanation became dysfunctional. Counseling consisted of reassurance that there was no doubt that the men would enjoy an active sex life after having recovered from the operation, despite not having a visible ejaculation (retrograde ejaculation).

Ileostomy and Colostomy

Any surgical intervention in the lower abdomen may result in the destruction of nerves or vessels during the surgical procedure, leading to erectile failure. Thus, inquiry should be made about sexual functioning after surgery. When a patient who has undergone lower abdominal surgery seeks help for erectile problems, information about the exact surgical procedure should be sought. A special problem exists in vascular surgery, where impaired vascular function (possibly causing erectile dysfunction) sometimes may be turned into a neurogenic erectile dysfunction after successful revascularization. This dysfunction is due to the simultaneous inevitable destruction of nerves involved in the mechanism of erection.

Men who have had ileostomy or colostomy operations may develop secondary erectile dysfunction because of their loss of self-esteem and the depression that may follow a surgical intervention of this kind. Sometimes it is possible by careful interview about the erectile pattern during the initial period after surgery to obtain the crucial knowledge that erections were normal during a short period after surgery. Then, when the patient returned home, he may not have been able to erect when he and his wife had to deal with the presence of the colostomy bag. This situation may easily develop into a vicious circle. The need for comprehensive information for patients who undergo major surgery that may change their appearance or functions is one of the most important tasks that the physician faces. Here, patients' clubs may be of value. As erectile function may be temporarily impaired after surgery (up to four to six months), it is necessary to support the patient during this period. If the patient is persistently dysfunctional, sex therapy should be instituted, preferably including the partner. If such therapy fails, penile implants may be considered as a treatment possibility.

Spinal Cord Injury

Modern medical technology has enabled more acutely and severely injured people to survive. The number of young persons with sequelae after trauma to the spinal cord has increased. Most of these patients are men.

One of the many problems that these men face is impaired sexual function, which may include complete or partial loss of erectile ability, ejaculatory disorders, and decreased fertility. During the period immediately following the injury, the functional effect of a cord lesion on sexual functioning is highly unpredictable. Often "spinal shock" may persist for months and postpone a slow return to the permanent condition, which is highly variable from patient to patient. Again, we urge that these matters be discussed with the patient at the appropriate time. It is the professional who should feel the way to this moment and not expect the patient to introduce the question of his future sexual functioning, as spinal cord injury is accompanied by a period of great anxiety and insecurity (Cole, 1979).

In general, it can be stated that erectile capability is maintained with higher lesions of the cord. In complete spinal cord transections, Bors and Comarr (1960) found that cervical lesions left 100% of the patients with an intact reflexogenic erection pattern. The occurrence of psychogenic erection in the absence of reflexogenic erection was reported in 27% of patients with complete lower motor-neuron lesions (reflex activity was absent in the sacral segments) by Bors and Comarr (1960) and in 7% by Cibeira (1970) in those patients with lesions lower than T12.

In patients with complete upper motor-neuron lesions (reflex activity present in the sacral segments), 95% had spontaneous erections, and 92% from penile stimulation. Of those who attempted coitus, 57% were successful. Only 1% could ejaculate. In incomplete upper lesions, 48% had psychic erections, 93% had spontaneous or reflex erections, and 25% could ejaculate. With complete lower neuron lesions, 12% had spontaneous erections and 15% were able to ejaculate. Pinprick perception, more than preservation of light-touch perception, in the sacral segments of patients with incomplete upper motor-neuron lesions, seems to be of significance prognostically for erection and ejaculation (Comarr, 1970).

Specialized treatment and psychic support are necessary to help the patient with spinal cord injury. A comprehensive discussion can be found in Cole (1979).

Other Neurological Etiologies of Erectile Dysfunction

Galen classified impotence as a "neurological paralysis," while some Arab physicians of the same period viewed it as a "neuropsychiatric disorder" (as reviewed by Mettler, 1947). Historically, there have been a variety of postulated central nervous system disorders regarded as "sexual neurasthenias." More recent neurological literature has documented that erectile failure may result from congenital malformations such as spina bifida, infections such as tabes dorsalis, degenerative problems such as Parkinson's disease, and possible autoimmune, or slow-growing, viral infections such as multiple sclerosis. Further, a series of temporal-lobe epileptics revealed that two-thirds had hyposexuality (Gastaut and Collumb, 1954). Focal lesions of the spinal cord due to tumor or trauma may, of course, also result in erectile dysfunction, as noted above. And it has recently been postulated that extreme stress or torture may produce sexual dysfunction (Lunde *et al.* 1981).

Neurological Sites

A possible site in man for potency was suggested by Meyers (1961), who reported loss of libido and erectile failure following bilateral interruption of an area of tissue approximately 1 × 1 × 2 centimeters made up of the ventral thalamic peduncle, the perifornical regions, and the dorsal medial hypothalamic nuclei. This intervention, directed at cutting the ansa lenticularis, was for the relief of bilateral hyperkinetic behaviors. However, Brindley (1981) noted that the precise area that induced the impotence is difficult to delineate from Meyers's report. The approach was through the corpus callosum, and a piece of fornix was sacrificed bilaterally; yet previously induced lesions in these areas in other patients had not caused impotence. Further, previous stereotaxic lesions intended to interrupt the ansa lenticularis bilaterally had also not produced impotence.

Penile erection may be induced in the squirrel monkey by electrical stimulation of a number of basal brain structures, including the septal region, the mammillary bodies, various thalamic nuclei, and the gyrus cinguli and the gyrus rectus (MacLean and Ploog, 1960, 1962). The hippocampus reportedly modifies the effect of stimulation in these areas.

Depth electrodes implanted in various areas of the brain, when stimulated, have been reported to yield erotic fantasies and sensation (Heath, 1964). Stimulation of the septal region or its principal outflow pathway, the medial forebrain bundle, have led to pleasurable sensations and sometimes penile erection. One patient had been severely depressed but discussed plans to seduce a girl within 15 min of septal region stimulation. When asked why he had changed the subject of conversation, he said, "The idea of the girl suddenly came to me." Other patients experienced strong pleasure associated with sexual feelings and orgasm following electrical or chemical stimulation of the caudate nucleus, the intralaminar thalamic nuclei, the midhypothalamus, the posterior hypothalamus, or the boundary of the hypothalamus and the tegmentum. However, in a more extensive series, during the course of stereotaxic stimulation under local anesthesia in 82 men, there were no reports of erection at 429 sites near the third ventricle (Sem-Jacobsen, 1966).

A unique case report is that of a man followed for 13 years who developed initial symptoms of progressive hypothalamic atrophy at age 39. The diagnosis was later confirmed by pneumoencephalography. Hypothalamic dysfunction included loss of libido and erectile failure. When symptoms of sexual dysfunction appeared, the patient was put on oral testosterone and then intramuscular long-acting testosterone. Neither had any effect on sex drive or potency. However, when he was put on a daily dose of 4.5 g of levodopa, his sexual interest and activity returned, along with a reduction of excessive drowsiness and sleeping.

When reevaluated at age 52, the patient had been on levodopa for four years, and the symptomatic improvement of sexual functioning had persisted. On two occasions, both placement on placebo and discontinuance of levodopa for several months produced loss of libido and erectile dysfunction. His serum levels of testosterone while he was on levodopa were in the normal range but dropped to subnormal when he was on placebo. The drop was more than twofold. His serum prolactin began to increase progressively after age 50 (after the onset of erectile failure) and remained elevated even though his sexual function returned with levodopa.

The authors (Kelts and Hoehn, 1978) suggested that since the patient did not respond to supplemental testosterone with an increase in libido or erectile capacity, damage to the hypothalamic areas sensitive to testosterone may have occurred. They pointed to the work of MacLean and Ploog (1960, 1962), in which electrical stimulation to these areas in squirrel monkeys resulted in penile erection.

They also suggested that the marked improvement in sexual performance and the decreased somnolence during therapy with levodopa may implicate dopaminergic and/or noradrenergic systems.

Epilepsy

The classic 1954 study of Gastaut and Collumb assessed sexual function in epileptics and showed that two-thirds of 36 temporal lobe epileptics were dysfunctional compared with patients who had other types of epilepsy and who were typically functional. Shortly after, 15 dysfunctional men, all of whom manifested evidence of temporal lobe damage, were reported by Hierons and Saunders (1966). They were between 31 and 48 years old at the onset of their sexual disturbance. Of these men, 12 had temporal lobe epileptic attacks at some time while they were dysfunctional, and 1 had major epilepsy only. In 3 of the men, dysfunction had preceded the development of epilepsy by six to nine months. The symptom complaint was either complete inability to obtain an erection or only occasional success, with a notable tendency to lose the erection once obtained. Sex drive was reported as "probably normal" in all cases. In 4 men, drugs brought the epilepsy under control and simultaneously improved their sexual functioning.

The Gastaut and Collumb study is often cited because of its finding that sexual losses in epileptic patients were confined to men with temporal lobe epilepsy. The more recent work of Blumer and Walker (1967) reports behavioral results from surgically removing the temporal lobe. This surgery was performed unilaterally in 11 temporal lobe epileptics with global hyposexuality. Four patients whose seizures were abolished by surgery recovered normal sexuality and two others showed clinical improvement but relapsed when their seizures recurred.

One hundred noninstitutionalized male epileptics, age 20 through 55, were reported by Saunders and Rawson (1970). Significant disturbances of sexual behavior occurred only in those patients with temporal lobe epilepsy. Here, 12 of 33 patients had some sexual disturbance. The patients were divided into the following groups: those who were dysfunctional but had a normal sex drive; those with both diminished sex drive and dysfunction; and those in whom antiepileptic drugs appeared to be causing a reduction in sex drive.

There were seven patients who became dysfunctional but continued to have a normal sex drive. They complained of either total inability to obtain an erection or failure to sustain an erection for more than a brief period. None of the patients were having frequent epileptic attacks except for one, in whom minor seizures occurred daily. For him, the onset of erectile failure coincided with the appearance of frequent temporal lobe seizures, although major seizures had occurred six months earlier. In another case, the onset of erectile failure coincided with the appearance of temporal lobe epilepsy. None of the patients in this group were thought to be taking "excessive" doses of anticonvulsants and, in fact, one patient was receiving none.

As for global hyposexuality, there were two patients in this group, and in each case, the epilepsy began after age 50. The hyposexuality, including impotence and loss of sexual interest, appeared at approximately the same time as the seizures. Prior sexual behavior had been normal. Neither patient was thought to be taking "excessive" anticonvulsant medication.

There was only one patient in whom there was good evidence that excessive anticonvulsants or the wrong type of anticonvulsant was responsible for the dysfunction. In this case, the patient was rendered drowsy under one type of medication, and when another was substituted, there was more general alertness and a restoration of "libido."

The authors contested other writers who have suggested that it is the anticonvulsant medication that is responsible for hyposexuality. They pointed to the fact that of their 67 patients with patterns of epilepsy other than temporal lobe, the anticonvulsant regimen was similar to the regimen of those with temporal lobe epilepsy. Yet, it was only with the latter type of seizure that a significant proportion of patients showed disordered sexuality.

Multiple Sclerosis

Sexual disturbances are reported to be common in the early symptoms of multiple sclerosis (Lilius *et al.*, 1976). In one series (Ivers and Goldstein, 1963), 26% of the male patients had erectile failure, and in another (Vas, 1969), 47% of the male patients had some impairment of erection in spite of the absence of marked neurological disability. Vas suggested that the impotence was caused by a spinal cord lesion in its lateral horn.

A questionnaire given to 115 males with multiple sclerosis by Lilius *et al.* showed that the patient's sex life was changed in 91% of these men. Either an "unsatisfactory" or a "finished" sex life was reported by 64%. Many patients in this state were in relatively poor physical condition. The duration of the disease was from 4 to 14 years. However, 14 other males, considered in relatively good physical condition, also had significant disturbances in erection. Interest in sexual intercourse decreased in 34% and was eliminated in an additional 22%. Capacity for erection was diminished in 80% and for ejaculation in 75%. While there was no correlation between the incidence of sexual disturbances and the duration of the disease, the occurrence of pyramidal tract symptoms and bladder dysfunction was of about equal frequency as that of sexual disturbance.

Thermoregulatory sweating-response tests in males with multiple sclerosis have been correlated with a variety of factors, including sexual functioning (Cartlidge, 1972). (The sweating response is a function of an intact autonomic nervous system.) The incidence of abnormal sweating responses was higher in patients with more severe multiple sclerosis but did not correlate well with the severity of disturbance of any one nonsexual function. Of the 20 male patients, 13 claimed to have normal potency, 5 had partial erectile failure, and 2 were totally impotent. All 7 with disorders of erectile function had impaired sweating. The 2 with total erectile failure had no sweating below the waist, and the 5 with partial failure had no sweating in the legs. The impotent patients did not appear to have more severe general disability due to their multiple sclerosis than those who were still potent.

Tobacco

A recent provocative report is that of Forsberg *et al.* (1979) on two patients 20 and 27 years of age, both smokers, who complained of erectile problems. Endocrine and general medical examination revealed nothing abnormal. Their systemic and penile blood pressures were within normal limits, but the ratio between flow acceleration in the penile and brachial artery was abnormal. After these patients discontinued smoking for a few days, the ability for erection reappeared both as morning erections and during sexual arousal. The flow acceleration curves changed dramatically in both cases, now being normal. One of the patients smoked only 10 cigarettes a day. Although the report is preliminary, it points to a hitherto unrecognized area that merits further investigation. Indeed, three more patients with the same condition have been subsequently reported by Forsberg and Olsson (1980).

Drugs

Controlled and objective studies of the effect of drugs on erection in normally functioning men are almost nonexistent. Alcohol has been studied (Chapter 8), and the effects of atropine, propranolol, and phenoxybenzamine have been mentioned.

Clinical trials in patients in whom a given drug is suspected of having a side effect on erectile function are few and difficult to perform. Our knowledge of this important aspect of drug side effects is therefore minimal. It is an area in need of considerable research.

Methyldopa, which depletes biogenic amines, is often cited as resulting in erectile dysfunction. It also increases the prolactin level. Thus, it cannot be said at which site its antierection effect might work. In a series of 10 normotensive men, 250-mg tablets were given 40, 30, 16, and 3 hr before a controlled laboratory study of erectile ability. In none was erection affected (Wagner *et al.* 1979). Acute experiments naturally do not exclude the possibility of other effects after the long-term use of a drug. Clonidine, another α-blocking agent used as an antihypertensive drug, is being repeatedly reported as causing erectile dysfunction. Fenfluramine—a sympathomimetic drug used in the treatment of obesity—has also been reported as causing erectile dysfunction. One explanation for this effect is a possible reinforcement of the antierectile sympathetic tone responsible for the contracted state of the smooth muscle of the cavernous bodies.

The reported effects of antipsychotic and antidepressant drugs are difficult to evaluate because of inadequate controls, concomitant psychiatric disorder, and inadequate biochemical correlates. This area is wide open for meaningful research.

Conclusion

Many common medical illnesses, in both the acute and the chronic phases, are interrelated with sexual functioning. The knowledgeable physician must understand these physiological interrelationships and be prepared to intervene where possible. The sympathetic physician must also understand the psychological interrelationships and be prepared for sensitive, detailed inquiry and possible counseling.

References

Abram, H. S., Hester, L. R., Sheridan, W. F., and Epstein, G. M. (1975). Sexual functioning in patients with chronic renal failure. *Journal of Nervous and Mental Disease*, *160*, 220–226.

Blumer, D., and Walker, E. (1967). Sexual behavior in temporal lobe epilepsy. *Archives of Neurology and Psychiatry*, *16*, 38–43.

Bommer, J., Ritz, E., Paso, E., and Bommer, G. (1979). Improved sexual function in male haemodialysis patients on bromocriptine. *Lancet*, *8*, 496–497.

Bors, E., and Comarr, A. E. (1960). Neurological disturbances of sexual function with special reference to 529 patients with spinal cord injury. *Urological Survey*, *10*, 191–222.

Brindley, G. S. (1981). Clinical practice in urology. In H. Margreve (Ed.), *Male Infertility*. Berlin: Springer Verlag.

Cartlidge, N. (1972). Autonomic function in multiple sclerosis. *Brain*, *95*, 661–664.

Chopp, R. T., and Mendez, R. (1978) . Sexual function and hormonal abnormalities in uremic men on chronic dialysis and after renal transplantation. *Fertility and Sterility*, *29*, 661–666.

Cibeira, J. B. (1970). Some conclusions on a study of 365 patients with spinal cord lesions. *Paraplegia*, *7*, 249–254.

Cole, T. (1979). Sexuality and the spinal cord injured. In R. Green (Ed.), *Human Sexuality: A Health Practitioner's Text (2nd ed.)*. Baltimore: Williams and Wilkins.

Comarr, A. E. (1970). Sexual function among patients with spinal cord injury. *Urologia Internationalis*, *25*, 134–168.

Forsberg, L., and Olsson, A. M. (1980). Presented at *Second International Conference on Vasculogenic Impotence*, Monaco, Oct. 8–12.
Forsberg, L., Gustavii, B., Hojerback, T., and Olsson, A. M. (1979). Impotence, smoking and β-blocking drugs. *Fertility and Sterility*, *31*, 589–591.
Fox C., Ismail, A., Love, D., Kirkham, K., and Loraine, J. (1972). Studies on the relationship between plasma testosterone levels in human sexual activity. *Journal of Endocrinology*, *52*, 51–54.
Friedman, J. M. (1978). Sexual adjustment of the post-coronary male. In J. LoPiccolo and L. LoPiccolo (Eds.), *Handbook of Sex Therapy*. New York: Plenum.
Gastaut, M., and Collumb, J. (1954). Étude du comportement sexual chez les epiléptiques psychomoteurs. *Annals Medico Psychologie*, *112*, 657–696.
Gittes, R. F., and Waters, W. B. (1979). Sexual impotence: The overlooked complication of second renal transplant. *Journal of Urology*, *121*, 719–722.
Green, R. (1979). *Human Sexuality: A Health Practitioner's Text (2nd ed.)*. Baltimore: Williams and Wilkins.
Hagen, C., Ølgaard, K., McNeilly, A. S., and Fisher, R. (1976). Prolactin and the pituitary gonadal axis in male uraemic patients on regular dialysis. *Acta Endocrinologica*, *82*, 29–38.
Heath, R. (1964). *The Role of Pleasure in Behavior* (R. Heath, ed.). New York: Harper & Row.
Hellerstein, H. K., and Friedman, E. H. (1970). Sexual activity in the post coronary patient. *Archives of Internal Medicine*, *125*, 987–999.
Hierons, R., and Saunders, M. (1966). Impotence in patients with temporal lobe lesions. *Lancet*, *2*, 761–764.
Ivers, R., and Goldstein, N. (1963). Multiple sclerosis: A current appraisal of symptoms and signs. *Proceedings Mayo Clinic*, *38*, 457–466.
Kass, I., Updegraff, K., and Muffly, R. B. (1972). Sex in chronic obstructive pulmonary disease. *Medical Aspects of Human Sexuality*, *6*, 33–42.
Kelts, K., and Hoehn, M. (1978). Hypothalamic atrophy. *Journal of Clinical Psychiatry*, *April*, 357–365.
Kolodny, R., Masters, W., Johnson, V., and Biggs, M. (1979). *Textbook of Human Sexuality for Nurses*. Boston: Little, Brown.
Levy, N. (1976). Coping with maintenance of hemodialysis. In S. G. Massry and D. Sellers (Eds.), *Clinical Aspects of Uremia and Dialysis*. Springfield, Ill.: Charles C Thomas.
Lilius, H., Valtonen, E., and Wikstrom, J. (1976). Sexual problems in patients suffering from multiple sclerosis. *Journal of Chronic Diseases*, *29*, 643–647.
Loew, H., Schultz, H., and Busch, G. (1975). Klinische Aspekte der Impotenz mannlicher Dauerdialysenpatienten. *Medizinische Welt*, *25*, 1651–1652.
Lunde, I., Rasmussen, O. V., Lindholm, J., and Wagner, G. (1981). Sexual and pituitary-testicular function in torture victims. *Archives of Sexual Behavior*, *10*, 25–32.
MacLean, P., and Ploog, D. (1960). *Federation Proceedings, American Society of Experimental Biology*, *19*, 288.
MacLean, P., and Ploog, D. (1962). Cerebral representation of penile erection. *Journal of Neurophysiology*, *25*, 29–40.
Massry, S. G., Goldstein, D. A., Procci, W. R., and Kletzky, O. A. (1977). Impotence in patients with uremia: A possible role for parathyroid hormone. *Nephron*, *19*, 305–310.
Mettler, F. (1947). In C. Mettler (Ed.), *History of Medicine*. Philadelphia: Blakiston.
Meyers, R. (1961). Evidence of a locus of the neural mechanisms for libido and penile potency in the septo-fornico hypothothalamic region of the human brain. *Transactions, American Neurological Society*, *86*, 81–85.
Nemec, E. D., Mansfield, L., and Kennedy, J. W. (1976). Heart rate and blood pressure responses during sexual activity in normal males. *American Heart Journal*, *92*, 274–277.

Neri, A., Aygen, M., Zukerman, Z., and Bahary, C. (1980). Subjective assessment of sexual dysfunction of patients on long-term administration of digoxin. *Archives of Sexual Behavior*, *9*, 319–326.
Saunders, M., and Rawson, M. (1970). Sexuality in male epileptics. *Journal of the Neurological Sciences*, *10*, 577–583.
Sem-Jacobsen, D. (1966). Depth electrography observations related to Parkinson's disease. *Journal of Neurosurgery*, *24*, 388–398.
Spark, R., White, R., and Conally, P. (1980). Impotence is not always psychogenic. *Journal of the American Medical Association*, *243*, 750–755.
Vas, C. (1969). Sexual impotence and some autonomic disturbances in men with multiple sclerosis. *Acta Neurologica Scandinavica*, *45*, 166–182.
Wagner, G., Zbytovsky, J., and Brindley, G. S. (1979). The effect of methyldopa, α- and β-blockers on penile erection in normotensive men. Presented at the meeting of the *International Academy of Sex Research*, Prague.
Wagner, G. (1976). *Physiological Responses of the Sexually Stimulated Male in the Laboratory*. 16 mm color film. Copenhagen/New York.
Wagner, G., and Brindley, G. S. (1978). The effect of atropine, α- and β-blockers upon human penile erection: A controlled pilot study. Presented at the *First International Conference for Vasculogenic Impotence*, New York.
Wolpowitz, A., and Barnard, C. N. (1978). Impotence after heart transplantation. *Suid-Afrikaanse Mediese Tydskrif*, *53*, 693.
Zarate, A., Canales, E. S., and Soria, J. (1972). Ovarian refractoriness during lactation in women: Effect of gonadotropin stimulation. *American Journal of Obstetrics and Gynecology*, *112*, 1130–1132.
Zohar, J., Meiraz, D., Maoz, B., and Durst, N. (1976). Factors influencing sexual activity after prostatectomy—A prospective study. *Journal of Urology*, *116*, 332–334.

CHAPTER 4

Diabetes Mellitus and Erectile Failure

GORM WAGNER, JANNIK HILSTED, AND
SØREN BUUS JENSEN

The first report of male erectile failure in diabetics was made by Rollo in 1798. Since then, many descriptions of the problem have been given, both in the preinsulin era (Nanuyn, 1906) and later. During the last 20 years, it has been established that erectile failure is a more common problem among diabetics than in the general population (Rubin and Babbott, 1958, Schöffling *et al.*, 1963; Ellenberg, 1971; Kolodny *et al.*, 1974; Jensen, 1981). Nearly half of younger diabetics report experiencing sexual dysfunction in epidemiological studies (Rubin and Babbott, 1958; Schöffling *et al.*, 1963; Ellenberg, 1971; Kolodny *et al.*, 1974; Jensen *et al.*, 1979). Diabetes mellitus is a typical example of the interplay between somatic and psychological factors.

Methodological Problems in Studying Sexual Dysfunction in Diabetes Mellitus

A critical review of the literature illustrates that our present knowledge is largely based on studies that lacked stringent methods regarding sexological data. Methodological necessities for such studies include the following:

1. The diabetes group should be *well characterized*: juvenile–mature onset, duration of the disease, age at onset of diabetes, and age at onset of sexual dysfunction. Long-term diabetic complications should be described. The criteria for inclusion or exclusion of subjects should be well defined.
2. A distinction must be made between complications of the disease and the possible consequences of treatment other than insulin.

3. Associated somatic diseases, psychiatric illness, alcohol abuse, and medications should be listed. It should be noted whether sexual dysfunction was associated with the administration of any medication.
4. Studies should be controlled and/or prospective.
5. Physiological methods should be used to quantify the degree of pathological conditions.
6. Stringent definitions of sexual dysfunction should be used. The dynamics of the symptoms, their variability, and the patient's subjective experience should be elaborated.
7. Sexological data should be presented in such a way that the conditions and instruments are clear-cut, so that these data may be adequately evaluated.

Strict definitions of the reduction of libido, careful sexological history, and supplemental observations given by the sexual partner are required. These data constitute part of the evaluation of the development of the erectile failure. They should be accompanied by information on the state of diabetic factors along with neurological, vascular, psychological, and hormonal factors.

Symptomatology

Most studies indicate that the frequency of sexual dysfunction in younger diabetic males is around 50% (Rubin and Babbott, 1958; Schöffling *et al.*, 1963; Kolodny *et al.*, 1974). In a study of insulin-treated diabetic male outpatients who were 26–45 years of age, compared with a matched control group from the general population, 44% of the diabetics versus 2.5% of the controls reported sexual dysfunction (Jensen, 1978). This difference was based on a significantly higher frequency of erectile failure among diabetics (34% versus 0%) and reduced libido (31% versus 2.5%). No difference in ejaculatory function was found between the groups.

The classic findings of diabetic erectile failure have been characterized as coital dysfunction (insidious), where libido is normal or even raised; a lack of morning erections; and a lack (partial or total) of erectile capacity during masturbation (Cooper, 1972). An analysis of these factors among diabetic patients with erectile dysfunction, supplemented by a psychological evaluation, was made by Jensen (1981). The symptom picture was of low diagnostic value in distinguishing between organic and psychogenic impotence. Even patients in whom other examinations (vasculogenic or neurogenic) showed a massive probability of an organic component in their sexual dysfunction revealed a marked superimposed psychological component.

During the last few years, several subclinical endocrine disturbances have been related to impotence. Whether these are a cause of or are caused by the erectile dysfunctional state is at this time impossible to evaluate. One example of this gray area has been demonstrated by Legros *et al.* (1978). Reaction to the oral glucose tolerance test was studied in 88 patients carefully diagnosed as having psychogenic erectile failure. Of these men 34% were found to have an abnormal glucose tolerance test (blood glucose $>$ 1.6 g/l at the peak and $>$ 1.2 g/l after 2 hr). Although their serum testosterone and LH levels were normal, as a group they were significantly different from a group of men whose glucose tolerance tests were normal.

Diabetic Factors

Several investigators have reported erectile dysfunction to be common early in the course of diabetes. At the onset of diabetes, psychological factors (alterations in way of life, social and occupational readjustments) and somatic factors (general disability due to insulin deficiency) are obvious. Most often, the patient regains his erectile capacity shortly after the institution of insulin therapy. Only a few remain dysfunctional (Rubin and Babbott, 1958). These patients have usually not been evaluated for vascular and neurological abnormalities, which may occur rapidly in some patients (Bennett *et al.*, 1975).

In one study (Jensen, 1978), 11% of diabetics reported retrospectively, that their sexual dysfunction started within the first year of diabetes, while more than 60% had had diabetes for more than five years at the onset of sexual symptoms. The age of onset of diabetes seems unrelated to sexual dysfunction in younger diabetic patients.

Most reports describe the diabetic erectile failure as having an insidious onset, but becoming total within a year from the first symptom. An ongoing prospective evaluation of erectile ability among 10 patients reporting marked erectile dysfunction revealed that none developed complete erectile failure within two years of observation (Jensen, unpublished).

The duration of manifest diabetes seems of lesser significance, whereas the age of the patient seems critical. Patients more than 40 years old report more problems than younger patients, irrespective of the duration of disease (Jensen, 1978). The rise in prevalence of diabetic complications with increasing age and the chronicity of diabetes (Pirart, 1977), coupled with the influence of increasing psychological problems, might explain these findings.

The Quality of Regulation

Patients have reported that they functioned better sexually with optimal biochemical regulation of their diabetes. Objective measures of the quality of regulation have not substantiated these findings, but stringent criteria for such quality are frequently not present. The insulin dose, the number of daily doses, and the type of insulin given seem, if sufficient for optimal regulation, unrelated to sexual dysfunction.

Some patients report fear of hypoglycemic episodes during sexual activity. One third of diabetic patients reported having experienced such episodes, but only 2.5% claimed them to be a common problem (Jensen, 1978).

Neurological Factors

Functional abnormalities of the nervous system can be demonstrated in the majority of diabetics after 10–15 years. These comprise changes in the somatic as well as in the autonomic nervous system.

Somatic nervous system abnormalities include loss of deep tendon reflexes and an increased threshold for the sense of vibration, especially in the lower extremities (Gregersen, 1969). In most studies, peripheral neuropathy has been significantly correlated with sexual dysfunction (e.g., Ellenberg, 1971).

Autonomic nervous system abnormalities include a decreased variation in heart rate during normal as well as forced respiration (sinus arrhythmia or beat-to-beat variation) (Figure 21). This finding is considered due to *parasympathetic* neuropathy (Hilsted and Jensen, 1979).

A decrease in plasma catecholamine level in the supine and standing positions, (Christensen, 1971) as well as during exercise (Hilsted *et al.*, 1979), probably reflects dysfunction of the *sympathetic* nervous system.

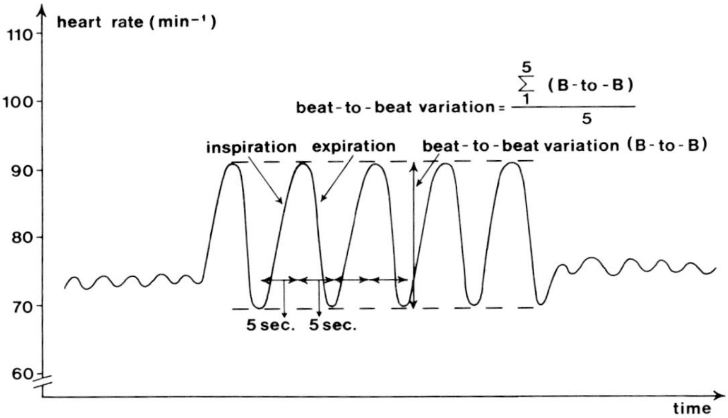

Figure 21. Calculation of beat-to-beat variation in heart rate during maximal respiration. Reduced values (10 beats/min) are regarded as being due to lesions in cardiac parasympathetic nerves.

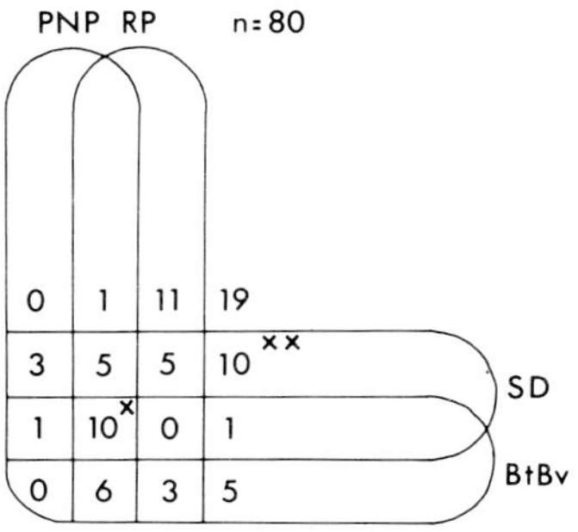

Figure 22. Diagram used for rapid analysis of 80 insulin-treated diabetic men (age group 26–45) as to incidence of sexual dysfunction (SD) and its relation to peripheral neuropathy (PNP), retinopathy (RP), and reduced beat-to-beat variation (BtBv). (x) denotes the group with all three pathological findings, while (xx) denotes the group with none of the pathological findings.

Most of the evidence of autonomic neuropathy as an etiological factor in diabetic erectile dysfunction is indirect. Direct functional studies of the autonomic nerves controlling erection have not hitherto been performed for methodological reasons. Urodynamic investigations have, in some studies, revealed a close relation to present erectile dysfunction (Ellenberg, 1971; Faerman *et al.*, 1971), while others (Frimodt-Møller, 1977) were unable to demonstrate such a relationship.

In 80 diabetic men, the interrelationship of sexual dysfunction and three different pathological findings (peripheral somatic neuropathy, retinopathy, and reduced beat-to-beat variation) was examined. Of these patients, 35 had a sexual dysfunction, and 26 of these 35 had erectile dysfunction. Only peripheral somatic neuropathy, and not retinopathy or reduced beat-to-beat variation, was found to be significantly correlated with sexual dysfunction (Figure 22). Interestingly, on autopsy, 5 previously diabetic males with erectile failure were found to have damaged automonic nerve endings under both light and electron microscopy (Faerman *et al.*, 1974).

Although it is not known which neurotransmitter(s) is involved in normal erection and tumescence, a single study of catecholamines has indicated a decreased content of norepinephrine in the cavernous tissue in diabetic men (Melman and Henry, 1979). Tissue was taken for analysis from four insulin-dependent diabetic men with erectile dysfunction who were planning to have a penile prosthesis inserted. A concentration of 59 ($\pm$28.4 SEM) pg/mg weight was found. This compared to 563 ($\pm$182.3) pg/mg in tissues of men with erectile function who required penectomy for other medical indications. In dysfunctional diabetics who were not insulin dependent no decrease in norepinephrine was observed. The interpretation of this finding is complicated since activity of the sympathetic nervous system is not usually assumed to be involved in the mechanism of erection. Yet the results indicate that the insulin-dependent dysfunctional male may have a defect in the sympathetic nervous system, possibly related to penile function.

Diagnostic Procedures (Neurological)

The required procedures include vibration threshold (Bio-Thesiometer) (Jersild and Lauritzen, 1957), tendon reflex examination, beat-to-beat pulse variation (Hilsted and Jensen, 1979), orthostatic blood pressure, and urodynamic evaluation, including the genital reflexes.

Vascular Factors (Angiopathy)

Long-term diabetic vascular changes affect both large and small vessels, that is, diabetic macro- and microangiopathy. These lesions are found in all organs, but only ocular, renal, cardiac, and lower-extremity changes are known to produce clinical symptoms (Lundbaek, 1959).

The functional consequences of diabetic microangiopathy include increased permeability and fragility of small vessels, while diabetic macroangiopathy is characterized by linear calcification in the large vessels of the extremities. Diabetic macroangiopathy could be at least partly responsible for the erectile dysfunction via arterial vascular insufficiency. Several techniques of penile blood-pressure measurement (Gaskell, 1971; Abelson, 1975) have demonstrated such a reduction. However, the patients in these studies appear to have been unrepresentative of diabetics in that a disproportionate number had documented vascular disease.

Observations of pathological conditions in the arterial bed supplying the penis were first reported by Rotter and Schurmann (1950) and later in a series of 15 diabetics with a mean disease duration of 13 years by Ružbarský and Michal (1977). Fibrotic lesions were found to predominate in the Ebner pads of the deep penile arteries as well as in the intima, although few thrombi were found. Calcification was found in the fibrotic pads and in the proliferated intima much more commonly in diabetic men than in a control group of deceased men matched for age. It was characteristic that the heaviest pathological involvement was in that portion of the penis below and behind the symphysis pubis and that pathological changes decreased in the direction of the glans (Table V). These findings can be taken as an indication of a positive correlation between arterial lesions and sexual dysfunction. There are, however, no data on the prior sexual function of the men studied post mortem.

In autopsy studies of cavernous tissue from five diabetics with erectile dysfunction, no microangiopathy could be demonstrated (Faerman *et al.*, 1974). Microangiopathy, measured by ophthalmoscopy of the retina, seems to be unrelated to sexual dysfunction (Ellenberg, 1971; Kolodny *et al.* 1974; Jensen, 1978).

In a mixed group of 47 insulin-treated and non-insulin-treated diabetic men with erectile failure of the average age 54 years, Jevtich (1980) compared Doppler examination of the penile arteries with cystometry and bulbocavernous reflex

Table V. Degree of Change in Penile Arterial Vessels in 15 Diabetic Men[a]

Age	Duration of diabetes (years)	Lumen	Calcification	Media	Pads + intima
39	(21)		++	+	+
47	(10)				+
54	(10)	+++	+++	+++	+++
60	(10)	+	+	+	++
60	(10)	++	+	+	++
61	(30)	++	++	+	++
63	(19)	++	+	+	++
63	(11)	+	++	+	++
64	(9)	+	+	+	++
65	(2)	++			++
66	(17)	+++	++	+	+++
67	(21)	+++	+++	++	+++
67	(5)	++	+	+	++
79	(10)	++	++	+	++
85	(11)	+++	++	+	+++

[a]Changes found were rated slight (+), moderate (++), or severe (+++) (cf. Table VI). Modified from Ružarský and Michal (1977).

latency time. While only 2 patients had normal findings in the Doppler examinations, 31 had normal cystometry and a normal reflex pattern. Of 29 patients with abnormal arterial findings, 60% did not have neuropathy. This particular study thus suggests that an arterial etiology is dominant in the diabetic male with erectile dysfunction. Retrograde ejaculation as a neurological disorder was a rare finding. Unfortunately, an adequate control group was lacking to give this new study greater significance.

Diagnostic Procedures (Vascular Factors)

Measurement of blood pressure, ophthalmoscopy, and clinical evaluation of lower-extremity circulation is required. Evaluation of renal function (serum creatinine and degree of proteinuria) is also necessary. In selected cases, arteriography may be indicated (see Chapter 8).

Hormonal Aspects

From endocrinological studies of 314 diabetics, Schöffling *et al.* (1963) concluded that erectile dysfunction should be seen as a hypogonadotropic hypogonadism and claimed that treatment with chorionic gonadotropin and testosterone had a positive effect on erection. However, the evaluation of androgenic function in other studies has not revealed an endocrine dysfunction other than diabetes (Ellenberg, 1971; Faerman *et al.*, 1971; Kolodny *et al.*, 1974; Jensen *et al.*, 1979). Measurements of estrogen and prolactin levels have generally shown no correlation with sexual dysfunction.

Diagnostic Screening

Serum testosterone (T), follicle-stimulating hormone (FSH), luteinizing hormone (LH), and prolactin (PRL) are indicated.

Psychological Aspects

Psychogenic erectile dysfunction has been reported to be rare in diabetics (Rubin and Babbott, 1958; Schöffling *et al.*, 1963; Kolodny *et al.*, 1974). However, recent investigations (Renshaw, 1976; Jensen *et al.*, 1979; Jensen, 1981) have suggested the importance of an interplay between psychological and organic factors. Renshaw has pointed to the risk of underestimating clinical depression in the diabetic. Anxiety, fear of future complications, the role of a chronically ill person with daily restrictions, anger ("Why me?"), reduced body concept, and fatigue are some problems involved (Jensen *et al.*, 1979). Furthermore, the disease may be used in the psychodynamic relationship of the partners ("the function of the dysfunction"). The same psychological problems as occur in nondiabetics may, of course, be seen in diabetics (see Chapter 6).

Diagnostic Procedures

Careful history taking including psychodynamic, social, and sexological factors, with data from the partner are indicated.

Other Aspects

Associated medical or psychiatric disease, alcohol abuse, and medication may influence sexual function. Thus, they should also be detailed.

Diagnosis and Treatment

Data collected by some of the recommended diagnostic procedures provide information on the etiology of diabetic erectile dysfunction. Figure 22 illustrates the relation of peripheral neuropathy and autonomic dysfunction (e.g., reduced beat-to-beat variation) and retinopathy to sexual dysfunction. An analysis of data from 80 insulin-treated diabetics, 26–45 years of age, revealed two major groupings of sexually dysfunctional diabetic patients. One group had all three complications and the other group had none.

Among diabetics reporting sexual dysfunction in an epidemiological study, only 20% wished to engage in sexological counseling or therapy. The diabetic men wanted to discuss their sexological problems in the diabetic clinic. They saw these problems as subaspects, among the other problems of being chronically ill (Jensen *et al.*, 1979).

Therefore, the diabetic clinic should be able to offer sexual counseling to the diabetic man and his partner. The staff should spend the necessary time discussing these matters and should be able to offer up-to-date information. Both partners should be involved. Good communication by itself might reduce the frequency of sexual dysfunction, especially where psychological problems are present. In some cases, the patients should be referred for sexological treatment.

If the superimposed psychological reactions are handled by careful treatment, even a massive organic involvement can be treated to the point where the sexual relationship is satisfying for the couple (Renshaw, 1976).

Hormones

Hormones should be offered only when a marked decrease in measured hormonal levels is found.

Surgery

Conservative treatment of erectile dysfunction is not always possible, and there may be a surgical solution. However, in the diabetic, as in other cases where surgery is considered, careful and long observation, possibly with some supportive psychotherapy, should precede the implantation of a penile prosthesis.

Conclusion

The high prevalence of diabetes in the population and the high incidence of erectile dysfunction in the diabetic make the diabetic a common patient. We do not know the etiology of this kind of sexual dysfunction, but we may assume that neurogenic, vasculogenic, and psychogenic etiologies are likely, either alone or in concert. The role of the physician treating the diabetic male is crucial in this context. Here, prophylactic work may prevent a subgroup of patients from developing serious sexual problems.

References

Abelson, D., (1975). Diagnostic value of the penile pulse and blood pressure: A Doppler study of impotence in diabetics. *The Journal of Urology*, *113*, 636–639.

Bennett, T., Hosking, D. J., and Hampton, J. R. (1975). Cardiovascular control in diabetes mellitus. *British Medical Journal*, *2*, 585–587.

Christensen, N. J. (1971). Plasma catecholamines in long-term diabetics with and without neuropathy and in hypophysectomized subjects. *Journal of Clinical Investigation*, *51*, 779–787.

Cooper, A. J. (1972). Diagnosis and management of endocrine impotence. *British Medical Journal*, *2*, 34–38.

Ellenberg, M. (1971). Impotence in diabetes: The neurologic factor. *Annals of Internal Medicine*, *75*, 213–219.

Faerman, I., Maler, M., Jadzinsky, M., Alvarez, E., Fox, D., Zilbervarg, J., Cibeira, J. B., and Colinas, R. (1971). Asymptomatic neurogenic bladder in juvenile diabetics. *Diabetologia*, *7*, 168–172.

Faerman, I., Glocer, L., Fox, D., Jadzinsky, M. N., and Rapaport, M. (1974). Impotence and diabetes. *Diabetes*, *23*, 971–976.

Frimodt-Møller, C. (1977). *Diabetic Cystopathy*. Copenhagen: Thesis.

Gaskell, P. (1971). The importance of penile blood pressure in cases of impotence. *The Canadian Medical Association Journal*, *105*, 1047–1051.

Gregersen, G. (1969). *Peripheral Nerve Function in Diabetes Mellitus*. Thesis, Aarhus University, Aarhus, Denmark.

Hilsted, J., and Jensen, S. B. (1979). A simple test for autonomic neuropathy in juvenile diabetics. *Acta Medica Scandinavica*, *205*, 385–387.

Hilsted, J., Galbo, H., and Christensen, N. H. (1979). Impaired cardiovascular responses to graded exercise in diabetic autonomic neuropathy. *Diabetes*, *28*, 313–319.

Jensen, S. B. (1978). Sexual dysfunction and diabetes mellitus. Thesis for the Gold Medal in Medicine, University of Copenhagen.

Jensen, S. B. (1981). Sexual dysfunction in younger insulin-treated diabetics: A comparative study. *Archives of Sexual Behaviour*, in press.

Jensen, S. B., Hagen, C., and Frøland, A. (1979). Sexual function and pituitary-gonadal axis in younger diabetic males. *Acta Medica Scandinavica Suppl.*, *624*, 65–68.

Jersild, M., and Lauritzen, E. (1957). Sensibilité vibratoire chez les diabétiques. *Le Diabète*, *6*, 237–241.

Jevtich, M. (1980). Erectile failure in diabetics. Presented at the *Second International Conference on Vasculogenic Impotence*, Monaco, Oct. 6–10.

Kolodny, R. C., Kahn, C. B., Goldstein, H. H., and Barnett, D. M. (1974). Sexual dysfunction in diabetic men. *Diabetes*, *23*, 306–309.

Legros, J. J., Mormont, C., and Servais, J. (1978). A psychoneuroendocrinological study of erectile "psychogenic impotence": A comparison between normal patients and patients with abnormal reaction to glucose tolerance test. In L. Carenza, P. Paucheri, and L. Zichelli (Eds.), *Clinical Psychoneuroendocrinology in Reproduction*. London: Academic Press.

Lundbaek, K. (1959). Late developments in long-term diabetic vascular disease. In K. Oberdisse (Ed.), *Diabetes Mellitus*. Stuttgart: Thieme.

Melman, A., and Henry, D. (1979). The possible role of the catecholamines of the corpora in penile erection. *The Journal of Urology*, *121*, 419–421.

Nanuyn, B. (1906). *Der Diabetes mellitus*. Wien: Holder.

Pirart, J. (1977). Diabète et complications dégénératives présentation d'une étude prospective portant sur 4400 cas observés entre 1947 et 1973. *Diabète and Metabolisme*, *3*, 97–107.

Renshaw, D. (1976). Impotence and diabetes mellitus. *Comprehensive Therapy*, *2*, 47–50.

Rollo, J. (1798). *John Rollo's Book: Cases of Diabetes Mellitus*. London: Dilly.
Rotter, W., and Schurmann, R. (1950). Die Blutgefasse des menschlichen Penis. *Virchows Archiv*, *318*, 352–393.
Rubin, A., and Babbott, D. (1958). Impotence and diabetes mellitus. *Journal of the American Medical Association*, *168*, 498–500.
Ružbarský, V., and Michal, V. (1977). Morphologic changes in the arterial bed of the penis with aging. *Investigative Urology*, *15*, 194–199.
Schöffling, K., Federlin, K., Ditschuneit, H., and Pfeiffer, E. F. (1963). Disorders of sexual function in male diabetics. *The Journal of the American Diabetes Association*, *12*, 519–527.

CHAPTER 5

Arteriosclerosis and Erectile Failure

GORM WAGNER AND PETER METZ

Forty years ago, the French surgeon Leriche (1940) described the occurrence of erectile impotence in patients with arterial thrombosis and occlusion of the aortic bifurcation. Although another description (Leriche and Morel, 1948) put strong emphasis on this finding, little notice was given to it until recent years.

Not before the pioneering work by the Czech surgeon Michal (Michal *et al.*, 1976) was the surgical treatment of the syndrome of Leriche and other arterial occlusive conditions considered in cases of erectile dysfunction. Michal demonstrated that it was possible to diagnose the arterial occlusion and its effect on normal blood supply to the cavernous bodies through phalloarteriography (Michal and Pospichal, 1978), and furthermore, that it was possible to reestablish the arterial supply surgically and regain erectile capacity (Michal *et al.*, 1973).

The frequency of erectile dysfunction caused by arterial disease is not known. It is documented that the dysfunction occurs increasingly with age (Kinsey *et al.*, 1948), and it is also known that arteriosclerosis increases with age. Although it is tempting to suggest a causal relationship, there is no scientific reason on which to base such an assumption.

From their studies of phalloarteriography, Ginestié and Romieu (1976) estimated that about 25% of all cases of erectile dysfunction are due to arterial insufficiency. In our studies among a group of men referred to a vascular service for evaluation of peripheral arterial disease, it was found by questioning that 40–50% complained of erectile dysfunction.

Insufficiency of the arterial blood supply during sexual stimulation resulting in erectile dysfunction is most often seen in patients over 40 years old, and arteriosclerosis is the predominant cause of occlusion of the arteries leading to the erectile tissue. Furthermore, arterial occlusions after pelvic fractures, arteriovenous anastomoses in the pelvic area, dysplasia of arteries, and sequelae of reconstructive surgery of the arteries of the legs have all been described as leading to erectile dysfunction.

Pathology

The arteriosclerotic changes that may influence erection are situated in the distal part of the aorta, in the common and internal iliac arteries, in the internal pudendal artery, and/or in one or more of the penile arteries.

Intermittent claudication and other peripheral ischemic symptoms are often present when the arterial occlusion is located in the aorta or in one or both of the common iliac arteries (Figure 23). As in other parts of the vascular system, the arteriosclerotic changes are most often initiated around bifurcations. The proximal as well as the distal part of the internal iliac artery may be affected. Another common site is where the internal pudendal artery passes the great sacrosciatic ligament. A further site is in Alcock's canal and at the division of the penile artery into the dorsal artery, the deep artery, and the artery of the bulb.

The dramatic increase in lumen required to create and maintain the high pressure in the cavernous spaces and the high flow to the glans necessitates a great elasticity and distensibility at the time when peripheral resistance should diminish. Thus, peripheral lesions in or around the muscular regulatory systems like the Ebner pads would be likely to cause impaired vascular reactions during sexual stimulation and could lead to erectile dysfunction. Only a few pathological studies of structural changes of the penile arteries have been undertaken. In their thorough study of the vessels of the penis, Rotter and Schürmann (1950) described eight cases with edema of the Ebner pads. All were due to acute vascular shock, surgical intervention in the abdominal cavity with complications leading to death,

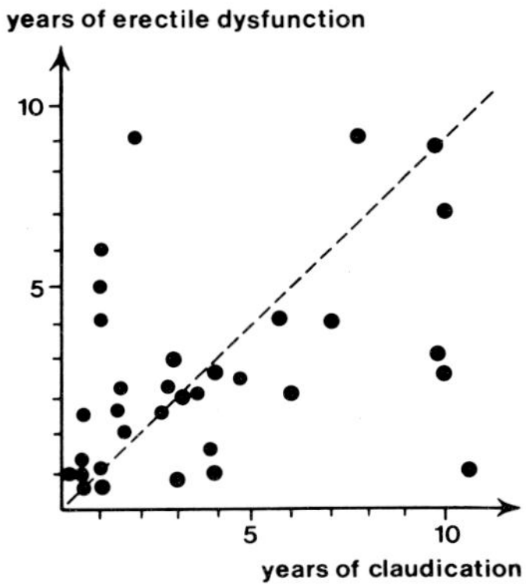

Figure 23. Relationship between durations of erectile dysfunction and intermittent claudication in 33 arteriosclerotic men, aged 39–69 years.

Table VI. Degree of Change in Penile Arterial Vessels in 15 Nondiabetic Men[a]

Age	Lumen	Calcification	Media	Pads + intima
19				
27				
38			+	+
42	+			+
44				+
47				+
52	++		+	++
55				+
60	+	+	+	+
61	+			+
64	++			++
65	+			++
66	++		+	+
67	++	+		+++
75	++	+	+	++

[a]Changes found were rated slight (+), moderate (++), or severe (+++) (cf. Table V). Modified from Ružbarský and Michal (1977).

or death due to complications of anesthesia. Changes were found in the arteries of men beginning at about the age of 50, and in one case at age 45. The helicine arteries appear to be affected by changes of the epithelioid cells, which show increased size with lipid droplets. In men in their 80s, fine calcifications can be noticed. The Ebner pads are frequently the sites affected. Generally, they are found to be enlarged, thereby decreasing the lumen and leading to increased resistance. Histologically, they appear to be sclerotic, and increasing hyalinization is associated with increasing age. These changes obviously hamper erectile function. The elastic fibers are few, and collagenous tissue dominates. Surprisingly, there may also be changes in the veins, with diminished smooth-muscle fibers, from about age 60. Increased collagenous tissue and a decrease of thickness of the walls of the veins have also been observed. Unfortunately, no histories of erectile function were recorded in any of these cases examined post mortem.

Post mortem histological material of 30 males from 19 to 85 years of age (mean 57) were recently investigated by Ruzbarsky and Michal (1977). Half had suffered from diabetes mellitus for a mean duration of 13 years. Table VI shows the findings in the 15 nondiabetic men. No information was obtained as to their erectile function. Pathology was found in the arterial tree to some extent in all men above 38 years. In the older men, larger segments of the dorsal artery were found to be partially or completely blocked by thrombi or fibroproliferative intima. In the deep artery, however, pathological changes in the Ebner pads dominated, while the artery of the corpus spongiosum rarely showed pathology. Fibrosis of the intima and replacement of the longitudinal smooth muscles by inelastic collagenous connective tissue were the most characteristic findings. In the media of the arterioles, fewer changes were found. Calcification was seen, dispersed or continuous, as deposits in the Ebner pads and in the proliferated intima. By histo-

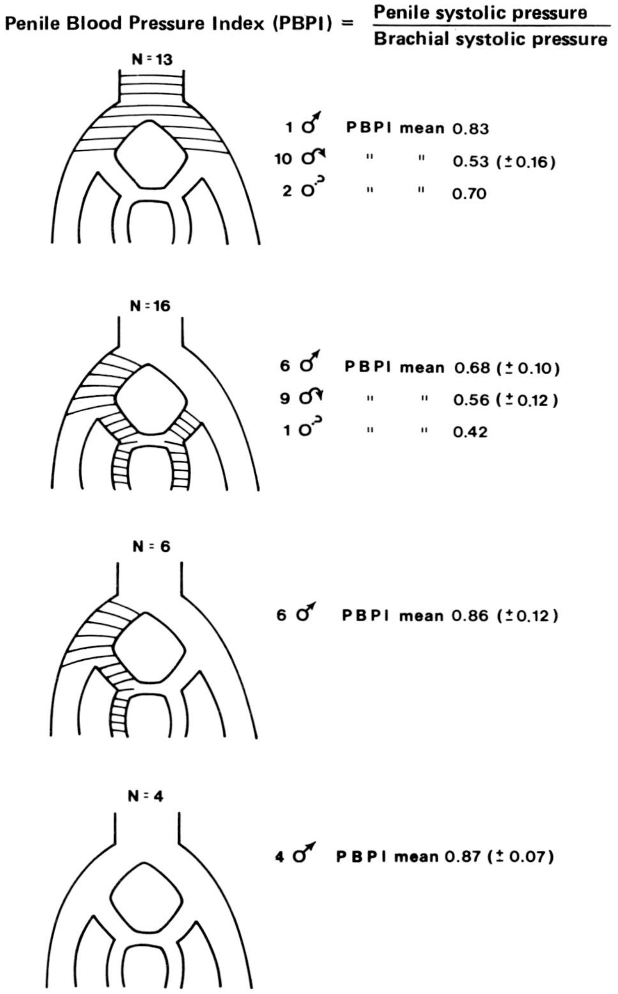

Figure 24. X-ray–localized lesions in 39 men with intermittent claudication. Penile blood pressure index (PBPI) is given as mean (± s.d.) in the 19 dysfunctional men, the 17 functional men, and the 3 men with no information on erectile function.

chemical techniques, delicate calcium deposits could be detected in cases where ordinary stained specimens appeared normal.

The microscopic lesions of the regulatory system and the subsequent narrowing of the arterial lumen necessarily must be followed by a decrease in function of the organ. As the findings seem related to age, they are in agreement with the decrease in potency reported in epidemiological studies like that of Kinsey and his co-workers. The changes in the local arteries show that a normal and sufficient blood flow may exist in the flaccid state but may not be sufficient to erect the penis. A gradual development of these changes is to be expected and may explain why the time necessary for erection extends with increasing age.

Arterial stenosis and occlusions from other causes may lead to low blood pressure, distal to the lesion in the smaller arteries of the penis in the flaccid state, and a lower filling pressure in the helicine arteries feeding the cavernous space. Because of insufficient pressure, erection may not occur when sexual stimulation takes place. Since a certain increase of flow rate is necessary and this too may be affected, maximum sexual stimulation, even for a long time, may fail to produce sufficient filling in spite of a normal intra-arterial pressure of the penile arteries.

There is not always a uniform relationship between penile blood pressure and arteriographic findings (cf. Figure 24), perhaps partly because of the development of collaterals. A uniform pattern is not found in these patients because of several factors. Penile blood-pressure measurement may not be a sufficient measure of blood flow rate or a sufficient index of the ability of blood to flow. Normal aorta–femoral angiography may not be sufficient to allow one to visualize the distal part of the internal pudendal and penile artery, and a man suffering from peripheral arteriosclerosis may be impotent from causes other than arterial insufficiency.

Symptoms

The symptoms of vasculogenic impotence due to arterial insufficiency differ only slightly from those due to other causes, partly because of secondary psychological aggravation and varied loss of libido. The erectile dysfunction starts gradually, now and then preceded for a period with problems of controlling ejaculation. Some patients have concomitant symptoms of arterial insufficiency in the legs, but in many cases, they consult their physicians solely for erectile dysfunction without intermittent claudication (see Figure 23).

The incompetent erectile capacity is usually constant, although differences in the power of the erotic stimulation and in demands for an erection may result in variation in erectile capacity. Thus, some patients are able to masturbate and ejaculate but not to have vaginal coitus, or they may be able to have coitus only in particular positions or with a particular partner.

The dysfunction often begins with an abnormal prolongation of the time taken to initiate and obtain full erection. Morning and spontaneous erections become weaker and occur less frequently, but both phenomena may continue to occur months or years after the initiation of the erectile dysfunction. The most common problem is to maintain the erection over any prolonged period, so that the patient must terminate coitus before ejaculation, although the initial erection was sufficient for vaginal intromission. Gradually, the erection becomes weaker and finally puts an end to coitus when intromission is no longer possible.

As a rule, the progression is slow, sometimes taking two to five years. Quite frequently, psychological problems intervene, such as performance anxiety, loss of self-confidence, and depression. These may cause a loss of sexual interest and may thereby put an end to sexual activity before the physiological erectile dysfunction itself brings about the end.

External Iliac "Steal Syndrome"

A special condition that may be easily confused with psychogenic impotence is the external iliac "steal syndrome." In this condition, the patient is able to achieve an almost normal erection but is not able to maintain it once coitus is initiated. The patient finds that his erection disappears immediately after he initiates coital movements. In some patients, gluteal pain occurs soon after. By modifying the coital posture from the prone position to a lateral or supine position in order to avoid large-scale muscle activity of the hip extensors, the problem may be corrected to some extent or may disappear. In most cases, the condition is seen in connection with more-or-less pronounced peripheral symptoms of arterial insufficiency, but it may precede intermittent claudication. The first example was described in 1978 by Michal, Kramář, and Pospichal; and the condition was also described later by Metz and Mathiesen (1979).

The pathogenesis of this condition is a concomitant restricted blood supply to the lower limbs and the pelvic area. Preoperative blood-flow measurements and angiographic studies have demonstrated that in cases of stenosis or occlusion in the common iliac artery, the blood flow through the internal iliac artery may reverse, the lower extremity being supplied by collaterals in the pelvic area. In occlusions of the distal part of the aorta, a collateral circulation may be established through the internal iliac arterial bed. In spite of these occlusions, the flow may be sufficient for the resting condition (flaccid state) and sufficient for an almost normal erection, but when dilatation of the arteries in the legs and/or the gluteal region occurs following muscle activation, blood flow to the pelvic area, including the cavernous bodies, drops and the erection stops. Soon after, the insufficient blood supply to the gluteal muscles may cause ischemic pain.

The characteristic symptoms, even in the absence of intermittent claudication, and the findings of reduced pulses or bruits in the groin should suggest this diagnosis. Without a physical examination, it can easily be interpreted as psychogenic.

Diagnosis

The diagnosis of arterial insufficiency as the cause in a case of erectile dysfunction must be based on the presence of occlusions in the arteries and a restriction of blood flow to the cavernous bodies. For the moment, measurement of the penile blood pressure is one of the most frequently used methods (see Chapter 8). It is predictable that a low arterial blood pressure in the penis or a low ratio of penile pressure to arm pressure will be followed by erectile failure, and it is unquestionable that significant differences can be found among groups of arteriosclerotic patients suffering from erectile failure, arteriosclerotic patients without failure, and normal potent men without arteriosclerosis. Nevertheless, the inability of the test always to predict whether a patient is potent, rendering its ability to diagnose an organic etiology for erectile failure uncertain, means that tests for arterial insufficiency are necessary (see Figure 25), just as distal blood-pressure

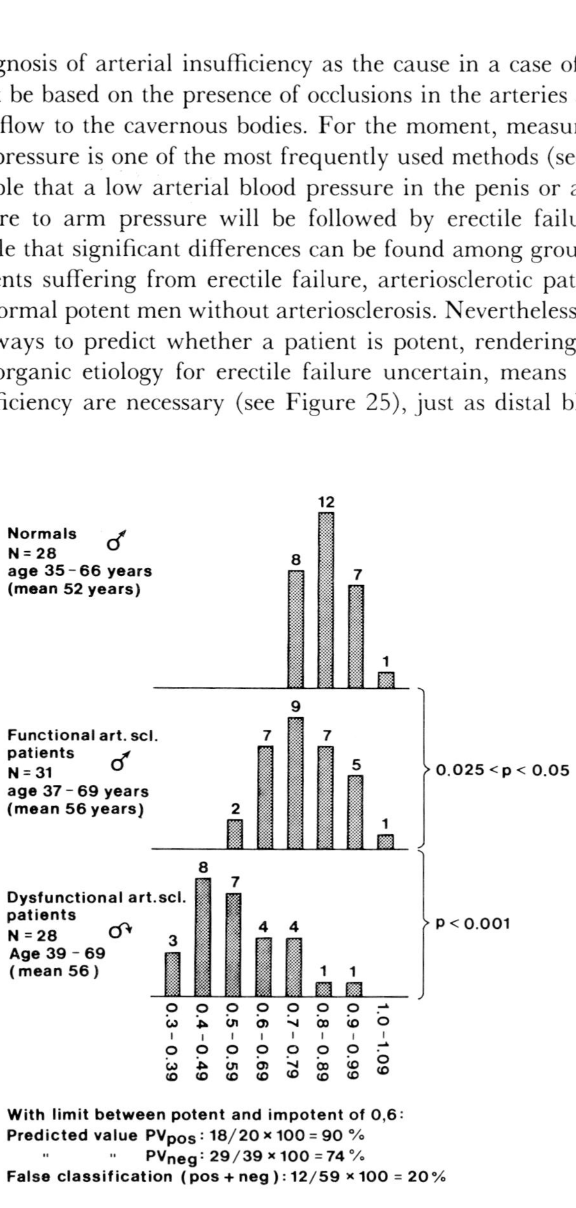

Figure 25. Penile blood pressure index (PBPI) in 28 normal, 31 functional arteriosclerotic, and 28 dysfunctional arteriosclerotic men in the same age range. There are significant differences between the groups, but there is considerable overlapping. The predictive value of the PBPI in dysfunctional arteriosclerotic men is indicated.

measurements used in the evaluation of arterial insufficiency in the legs are a useful tool for referring to groups of patients and controls before and after an operation, but not for predicting the degree of disease in any one individual.

The appearance of the pulse curve in the penile arteries and the acceleration of flow velocity obtained by the directional ultrasonic Doppler technique have also been employed in the evaluation of penile blood flow (Chapter 8, p. 100). Postischemic reactive hyperemia in the penis has been used as a diagnostic test measuring the penile blood pressure and pulse waveform in a group of dysfunctional and functional men after arterial closure by a cuff around the root of the penis. No difference in the reactive pattern was found (Kempczinski, 1979). Current investigations measuring the disappearance of a tracer from the cavernous body in the postischemic phase may provide more precise information about the flow conditions of the erectile tissue in the flaccid state.

The definitive diagnosis of an arterial lesion, but not necessarily evidence that the erectile dysfunction is caused by this, depends on the demonstration of stenosis or occlusion on radioangiograms. Visualization of the penile arteries is difficult and requires bilateral selective internal iliac arteriography. Different methods of obtaining optimal angiograms have been suggested, but it is not evident that one is better than another. The procedure is not without risk when bilateral catheterization of the femoral arteries is performed. It is therefore obvious that the procedure should be used only when there are reasons to believe that the dysfunction is vasculogenic and can be treated.

In a recent critical work, Buvat *et al.* (1979) studied 31 dysfunctional men on whom arteriography was performed in an effort to discover the relation between psychological patterns of behavior and the development of a documented dysfunction. The age range was 25–57 years (mean 44 years). All these men complained of an inability to achieve the degree of erection necessary for coitus in more than 50% of their attempts. An interview, a clinical examination, and a complete metabolic and endocrine investigation eliminated every organic etiology other than the vasculogenic. Arteriography was performed and a set of scores was applied to the radiographic findings in order to quantify the degree of arterial lesion. No investigations were undertaken of regulation of arterial blood flow or, specifically, of abnormal drainage from the cavernous bodies. Arteriography showed abnormalities in 75% of the men. No statistically significant difference could be detected in regard to psychological or behavioral abnormalities between the group with radiological pathology and the group with normal arteriography. The only anamnestic difference was the ability to keep an erection for more than five minutes, which none of the men with demonstrable arterial lesions were able to do. This criterion can be used for the selection of patients, as no abnormalities in the arteries were found in the 25% who were able to maintain an erection for more than five minutes.

None of the men were offered surgical therapy, although they were offered vasodilators or psychotherapy or given a placebo (in a noncontrolled way). One third (42% with mild abnormalities and 22% with severe abnormalities) regained a "satisfactory sex life" after 6–12 months. Of the 8 men with normal arteriography, 6 also attained a better sexual life. The researchers concluded that surgical intervention should not be undertaken hastily after the diagnosis has been made. The conclusion that surgery should be postponed is obviously correct. Patients should be followed for some period. However, there is no adequate explanation of why the men subjectively got better. It is known that collaterals may develop after localized occlusions, and such a development cannot be ruled out in these cases, as no control arteriography was performed.

The decision to undertake a surgical treatment of arterial insufficiency is influenced by several factors. The age of the patient, his health, other arteriosclerotic manifestations, and his partner's conception of the situation must all be considered. We asked a group of dysfunctional patients with peripheral arteriosclerosis of the legs whether they wanted a separate surgical intervention for impotence; 50% immediately stated that they would accept such an offer, while another 25% wanted to discuss the question with their spouse before accepting. (It should be mentioned that these men were covered by a free medical-care system.) In patients consulting a physician only for impotence, the percentage accepting may be expected to be higher.

Some patients, however, want only to be given a medical diagnosis and to be able to assure themselves and their partner that the dysfunction has an organic cause. Other patients can be helped by knowledge of the pathogenesis, by instructions about alternative sexual activities, or by relief from performance anxiety. The possible surgical interventions are discussed in Chapter 12.

Conclusion

A large group of arteriosclerotic patients with intermittent claudication experience erectile dysfunction. In some cases, this is the first symptom of an arterial lesion. Penile blood pressure, Doppler flow-velocity, and postocclusive blood flow measurement are diagnostic tools that indicate arterial pathology. Only radiological arteriography reveals the localization of the lesion. A special condition is the external iliac steal syndrome; this can be recognized through careful history taking.

References

Buvat, J., Dehaene, J. L., Lemaire, A., and Buvat-Herbaut, M. (1979). Erectile impotence by or with arterial abnormalities—Lack of correlation between arteriography and physiological disturbance. Presented at the *V World Congress of Sexology,* Mexico.

Ginestié, J-F., and Romieu, A. (1976). L'Exploration radiologique de *l'impuissance.* Paris: Maloine s.a. editor.
Kempczinski, R. F. (1979). Role of the vascular diagnostic laboratory in the evaluation of male impotence. *American Journal of Surgery, 138*, 278–282.
Kinsey, A., Pomeroy, W., and Martin, C. (1948). *Sexual Behavior in the Human Male.* Philadelphia: W. B. Saunders.
Leriche, R. (1940). De la reséction du carrefour aorticoiliaque avec double sympathecromie lombaire pour thrombose arteritique de l'aorte; le syndrome de l'oblitération terminoaortique par arterite. *Presse medicale, 48*, 193–206.
Leriche, R., and Morel, A. (1948). The syndrome of thrombotic obliteration of the aortic bifurcation. *Annals of Surgery, 127*, 193–206.
Metz, P., and Mathiesen, F. R. (1979). External iliac "steal syndrome" leading to a defect in penile erection and impotence. *Vascular Surgery, 13*, 70–72.
Michal, V., and Pospichal, J. (1978). Phalloarteriography in the diagnosis of erectile impotence. *World Journal of Surgery, 2*, 239–248.
Michal, V., Kramář, R., Pospichal, J., and Hejhal, L. (1973). Prima tepenna anastomoza na corpora cavernosa penis v lecbe erectivni impotence. *Rozhledy v chirurgii, 52*, 587–591.
Michal, V., Kramář, R., Pospichal, J., and Hejhal, L. (1976). Gefässchirurgie erectiver Impotenz. *Sexualmedicin, 5*, 15–20.
Michal, V., Kramář, R. and Pospichal, J. (1978). External iliac "steal syndrome." *Journal of Cardiovascular Surgery, 19*, 255–257.
Rotter, W., and Schürmann, R. (1950). Die Blutgefasse des menschlichen Penis. *Virchows Archiv, 318*, 352–397.
Ružbarský, V., and Michal, V. (1977). Morphological changes in the arterial bed of the penis with aging. *Investigative Urology, 15*, 194–199.

CHAPTER 6

Psychological Theories of Erectile Failure

RICHARD GREEN

Introduction

Impotence. Erectile failure. Why? While there is no shortage of soft speculation, there is a mere modicum of hard evidence. Theories, sometimes cloaked in authoritarianism, have existed for centuries. More recently, psychological studies, often overgeneralized, have accreted some insights, and modern endocrine and vascular technologies have identified some previously idiopathic or misdiagnosed causes.

This chapter highlights the most commonly suggested psychological etiologies of erectile failure. The goal is not to give exhaustive coverage but to set this vantage point in perspective, to be viewed alongside those of a primarily neurogenic or vasculogenic nature.

Historical Notes

Hippocrates noted in about 400 B.C. that constitutional elements were important in determining sex drive. He also suggested that "preoccupation with male affairs" and "lack of womanly attractiveness" were causative factors behind impotence (translated by W. Jones, 1948). A congenital variety of impotence was included in an ancient Hindu classification of sexual disorders, and a Hindu medical text suggested that one kind of impotence was due to "excessive venery" (Wise, 1845). Wong and Wu (1936) quoted a Chinese physician of the Golden Period of 1000 B.C. to A.D. 1000 who suggested that women be approached in "strict moderation." A book that by 1730 was published in its 18th edition (Tissot, 1764) indicted masturbation as inducing insanity, blindness, and impotence.

The classic *Golden Bough* (Frazer, 1955 printing) cites examples from earliest times when temporal and spiritual power were combined in the priest–king. The king's health and strength, and particularly his sexual potency, were believed to affect the harvest directly. The king's failure to satisfy his numerous consorts sexually was regarded as a sign of societal decay that could be remedied only by the king's execution.

Erectile failure was frequently believed to be the result of a divine curse, examples of which are found in the Satyricon of Petronius, in the Histories of Herodotus, and in the Bible (Genesis 20:1) (cited by Cooper, 1969). In the Middle Ages, erectile failure was frequently attributed to sorcery, when it was known as *ligature.* Then it was believed to have been inflicted by a witch's tying knots in a cord or a strip of leather and hiding it. Impotence persisted until the cord was discovered and the knots were untied.

In the United States, Dr. Benjamin Rush, a signer of the U.S. Declaration of Independence, noted in 1830 that "undue or a promiscuous intercourse with the female sex, or . . . onanism . . . produces seminal weakness, impotence" (p. 347). The 1858 version of Copland's *Medical Dictionary,* under the heading of "moral or mental impotence," listed fear of incapacity, not being loved, timidity, shame, disgust, hatred, jealousy, suspense, and terror as causes.

More Contemporary Writings

In the early 20th century, Freud believed that "neurasthenia" in males had at its root masturbation, the frequency of which ran parallel with the frequency of neurasthenia. When this continued for a long time, it impaired potency (*Collected Papers,* Vol. 110, 1950). Freud also suggested that disgust, resulting from a child's discovery that his mother has no penis, could produce impotence (*Collected Papers,* Vol. 110, 1950), and his grand biographer, Jones (1919), stressed the male's negative attitude toward the female's genitalia, replete with repulsion and disgust because of their association with excretory functions.

Freud stated that some homosexual men were unable to perform heterosexual coitus because of an intense fixation on their mothers and an identification with them that resulted in a search for young men resembling themselves (*Standard Edition,* Vol. 7, 1953). And the same factors that evolve toward a homosexual orientation have been proposed by Fenichel (1945) as making the male impotent with females (again, as with Freud, a circular argument which assumes that a homosexual orientation and heterosexual impotence are equatable).

Impotence with only a loved female was also described by Freud. In 1912, he wrote of a characteristic type of erectile failure in which the male loves his wife dearly and is impotent with her, although not with other females. Freud pointed out that in the emotional development of the boy, affectionate and love feelings for the mother develop much earlier than the sensual erotic feelings arising at puberty. If the newer sensual feelings become attached to incentuous fantasies, the result is impotence. The requisite for psychosexual maturity is that the older affectionate feelings be freed from the forbidden mother and fused with the newer sensual ones, with both becoming attached to the loved "object"—the wife. It was Freud's belief that the degree of fusion determined the degree of potency. Referring to incomplete fusion, he poignantly said, "Where they love, they do not desire and where they desire they cannot love. They seek objects which they do not need to love" (Freud, 1912, p. 183). This theory has been popularized as the "madonna–whore syndrome," where men are able to have intercourse with prostitutes, but not with wives.

Other psychoanalytic writings have traditionally stressed castration anxiety (Fenichel, 1953; Jones, 1919; Menninger, 1935; Stekel, 1927). Fear of punishment for observing parental sexual activity, fear of worry over financial matters, fear of disease, fear of pregnancy, and fear of inflicting injury on the partner have also been suggested (Podolsky, 1953). The *vagina dentata* theory made its mark! Here, the male fantasizes that the vaginal orifice acts as a castrating mouth with teeth. This fear leads to the inability to effect vaginal penetration.

"Coital anxiety" has more recently been seen by Cooper (1969) as a factor in a series of patients. This includes fear of failure, fear of being seen as sexually inferior by the partner, and fear of ridicule. However, Cooper concluded that cause and effect were not proved.

Hostility and resentment have also been linked with erectile failure (Wolberg, 1948; Hastings, 1963). A bipolar component of hatred was postulated as essential to every love by Stekel (1927) over a half century ago, and has been elegantly elaborated and extended by Stoller (1979).

A variety of personality factors have been implicated in the search for etiology. Feelings of inferiority and undue sensitivity to criticism have been suggested (Gutheil, 1959). Males with psychogenic erectile failure have been reported as excessively shy, submissive, withdrawn, and unduly sensitive to criticism, particularly relating to their physical appearance (el-Senoussi *et al.*, 1959). In another study, Cooper (1967) found that the most common personality type was "an hysterical personality abnormality," frequently manifesting as immature, attention-seeking, and manipulative behavior. Often the potency disorder was seen as part of a "punitive" behavior pattern between the spouses.

Inhibitory factors stemming from religion were suggested by Kinsey *et al.*, (1948) and then by Masters and Johnson (1970). Kinsey also suggested that ignorance of the normal biological variation in sexual performance was associated with impaired potency, with the male victims feeling that they were not living up to a sexual stereotype. Other researchers have suggested that childhood sexual misinformation, used to discourage masturbation, can lead to later sexual inhibition (Allen, 1962)—one example being "a drop of semen is equal to a pint of blood." Much of this latter type of "information" has persisted until "contemporary" times. The 1945 version of the United States *Boy Scout Manual* warned young males against "wasting their vital fluid."

Severe depression, particularly of an "endogenous" type, is often associated with erectile dysfunction. Indeed, in the widely used Hamilton Rating Scale of Depression, loss of sexual interest is a symptom that contributes to the total depression score. Worse yet is the "koro syndrome," a condition that manifests itself as great anxiety over the belief that the penis is shrinking. Not surprisingly, erectile failure is a common accompaniment (Yap, 1965).

Potency during advanced age is a controversial topic. Kinsey and his coworkers (1948) documented enduring percentages of males potent into advanced decades and concluded that "psychosocial factors" were prominent in the fall-off of sexual interest in many aging males. By this, they meant the men become satiated with their sexual partners of several decades. Support of this view is offered by the phenomenon that older males, dysfunctional with their wives, may be functional with young, new girlfriends. However, Cooper (1967) found that such improvements were rather short-lived and that sexual performance waned to previous levels within a few months with the new partner. (Some males, however, attempt to find sequential new partners for "perpetual potency.") Masters and Johnson's (1966) research stresses that although physiological changes in the male sexual-response cycle do evolve with age, erectile failure is not inevitable and can be ascribed to psychosocial factors.

Another pattern of erectile failure is the loss of erection after vaginal penetration but prior to orgasm and ejaculation (Hastings, 1971). Here, the dysfunction is seen as relating to feelings of guilt, fear of discovery in an illicit affair, or fear of pregnancy. Another common cause is also described by Hastings: the male finds his partner to be unresponsive. A casual remark during coitus about a household problem may often cause the erection to falter by making the male aware that the partner's mind is elsewhere. As Stafford-Clark (1954) noted,

> Owing to the very nature of her anatomy, a female can permit intercourse even though she is in no way inclined for it and not in the least interested in it. She can permit it physically while she is worrying about the housekeeping or about the children or thinking of other things or even another person, with her mind perhaps loaded with anxious or even guilty preoccupations of which her husband or lover may know nothing. On the other hand, a man is very rarely able to do anything like this. He cannot command his own erection; it is something which happens to him when he is in a certain emotional frame of mind . . . in one sense the man is, so to speak, on trial in a sexual situation. (p. 399)

Masters and Johnson, in their pioneering 1970 text, stated that of their 213 cases, less than 10% manifested physiologically based erectile dysfunction. They listed several psychogenic etiological factors: secondary dysfunction following premature ejaculation, secondary dysfunction following an acute alcoholic episode, maternal dominance leading to faulty male identification, paternal dominance leading to a faulty image of the female and feelings of inferiority, religious teaching of the sinfulness of sex, and a homosexual orientation. The assertion that approximately 85% of impotence is psychogenic was later made by Kaplan (1974, 1975). However, she also commented, "it may be speculated that patients who develop impotence are burdened by an especially reactive vasocongestive genital system. Whether experiential or constitutional factors are more influential in creating this vulnerability is purely conjectural" (Kaplan, 1974, p. 265).

The *fear of failure* following a single episode of erectile failure has been stressed as resulting in continuing sexual dysfunction; there is "fear of performance." This causes more episodes of dysfunction, and a self-perpetuating cycle of fear and dysfunction is established. As Masters and Johnson (1970) noted,

> Fear of inadequacy is the greatest known deterrent to effective sexual functioning, simply because it so completely distracts the fearful individual from his or her responsivity by blocking reception of sexual stimuli either created by or reflected from the sexual partner. (p. 12)

The characteristic symptom of psychologically caused impotence, underscored by Hastings (1971), is that it is *selective* in nature: it occurs under one set of circumstances but not under another. Hastings also suggested an "impotence of inexperience," where the "healthy" young male at the outset of his sexual life is troubled by impotence or premature ejaculation until he has gained experience. This reaction is due to a feeling of ineptness, a fear of hurting the female, an inability to reconcile a loved female with sexual passion, feelings of guilt and wrongdoing, and fear of pregnancy. As a prophylactic, Hastings advised that it is good to reexamine, prior to marriage, some of the old biases, prejudices, and notions about sexuality carried from one's childhood training.

Men suffering from primary erectile failure often come from sexually repressed or religiously orthodox family backgrounds where sex was not discussed or else was treated as sinful and immoral, according to Marmor (1976). Further, they often have abnormally close relations with seductive mothers and thus develop strong unconscious feelings of incest guilt during attempts at heterosexual functioning.

Apart from specific mother–son relationship factors, any life factors that make a male unusually fearful of intimacy, inordinately immature, inadequate, or deeply distrustful, fearful, or hostile to women may render him impotent (Marmor, 1976). Factors contributing to such reactions may include a rejecting or derogating mother or father, dominant older siblings, intense parental quarreling, feelings of being physically unattractive or uncoordinated, and rejection by peers. Added to such critical early-life experiences is the "cultural ambience," particularly in middle-class families, that makes sexual intercourse a difficult process to achieve in reality because it is surrounded by taboos and societal restrictions. Frequently, young males making their initial attempts at coitus in the back seat of a car or in a girlfriend's living room, settings frought with danger of discovery, may be so beset with anxiety that no erection occurs. With failure goes the fear of failure and the greater possibility of subsequent failure. When the initial erectile failure is triggered by the nonresponsiveness of the initial female partner, preexisting guilt and anxiety may be intensified. But the factor considered to be the most frequent of all is the preexisting pattern of premature ejaculation. This leads to increasing fears of sexual failure and secondary impotence (Marmor, 1976).

Etiology as Revealed by Treatment

A case study in which hypnotherapy was used to treat erectile dysfunction was described by Deabler (1976). After hypnotic induction, the patient was told to imagine himself in a sexual situation with his wife. Through an ideomotor technique, communication was established for mental images that appeared to relate to his sexual behavior. Indicators of sexual inhibition were elicited. Thus, some conscious factors were communicated.

Three layers of unconscious inhibitory factors were uncovered: first, there were early vivid memories of punishment for masturbation. This punishment had been administered by his mother. There was some improvement in sexual functioning after uncovering and reinterpreting the masturbatory punishment memories. An additional unconscious layer was early adolescent memories of his mother sternly lecturing him about the evils of sex and strongly admonishing him to stay away from girls. The third layer was a repressed image of an adolescent memory in which he would visualize his mother naked while he masturbated. There was a close physical resemblance between both of his wives and his mother. Through hypnotherapy, fear and anxiety related to sex were alleviated, and a positive attitude toward sex, particularly toward his wife, was suggested. A disidentification between wife and mother was made. The sexual dysfunction ceased.

Conclusion

These theories are varied. They are nonspecific. Some have a common fit; others are unique. Some have face validity; others appear exotic. Small wonder that we have moved to surgical technology, where phenomena can be quantified, where precision is paramount. But, psychogeneticists, do not abandon hope. The brilliant success on today's operating table may fade as quickly as yesterday's posthypnotic suggestion.

References

Allen, C. (1962). *Textbook of Psycho-Sexual Disorders*. London: Oxford University Press.

Cooper, A. (1967). Unpublished M.D. thesis, University of Bristol.

Cooper, A. (1969). Outpatient treatment of impotence. *Journal of Nervous and Mental Disease, 149*, 360–371.

Deabler, H. (1976). Hypnotherapy of impotence. *American Journal of Clinical Hypnosis, 19*, 9–12.

Fenichel, O. (1945). *The Psychoanalytic Theory of Neurosis*. New York: W. W. Norton.

Fenichel, O. (1953). *Collected Papers: First Series*. New York: W. W. Norton.

Frazer, J. (1955). *The Golden Bough*. London: Macmillan.

Freud, S. (1912). On the universal tendency to debasement in the sphere of love. In *Standard Edition of the Complete Psychological Works of Sigmund Freud,* Vol. 11 (J. Strachey, Ed.). London: Hogarth Press.

Freud, S. (1950). *Collected Papers*. Vol. 110. London: Hogarth Press.

Freud, S. (1953). *Three Essays on the Theory of Sexuality*. In *The Standard Edition of the Complete Psychological Works of Sigmund Freud,* Vol. 7 (J. Strachey, Ed.). London: Hogarth Press.

Gutheil, E. (1959). Sexual dysfunction in men. In S. Arieti (ed.), *American Handbook of Psychiatry*. New York: Basic Books.

Hastings, D. (1963). *Impotence and Frigidity*. London: Churchill.

Hastings, D., (1971). *A Doctor Speaks on Sexual Expression in Marriage*. Boston: Little, Brown.

Jones, E. (1919). *Papers on Psychoanalysis*. New York: Wood.

Jones, W. (Trans.). (1948). *Airs, Waters, Places,* XVII–XXII (ca. 4th century B.C.), Vol. 1. London: Heinemann.

Kaplan, H. (1974). *The New Sex Therapy*. New York: Bruner/Mazel.

Kaplan, H. (1975). *The Illustrated Manual of Sex Therapy*. New York: Quadrangle.

Kinsey, A., Pomeroy, W., and Martin, E. (1948). *Sexual Behavior in the Human Male*. Philadelphia: W. B. Saunders.

Marmor, J. (1976). Impotence and ejaculatory disorders. In B. Sadock, H. Kaplan, and A. Freedman (Eds.), *The Sexual Experience*. Baltimore: Williams and Wilkins.

Masters, W., and Johnson, V. (1970). *Human Sexual Inadequacy*. Boston: Little, Brown.

Menninger, K. (1935). Impotence and frigidity from the standpoint of psychoanalysis. *Journal of Urology, 34*, 166–188.

Podolsky, E. (1953). *What You Should Know about Sexual Impotence*. New York: Cadillac.

Rush, B. (1830). *Medical Inquiries and Observations upon the Diseases of the Mind*. Philadelphia: Grigg.

el-Senoussi, Coleman, D., and Jaubei, A. (1959). Factors in male impotence. *Journal of Psychology, 48*, 3–46.

Stafford-Clark, D. (1954). The etiology and treatment of impotence. *Practitioner, 172*, 397–404.

Stekel, W. (1927). *Impotence in the Male*. New York: Liveright.

Stoller, R. (1979). *Sexual Excitement*. New York: Pantheon.

Tissot, S. (1764). *L'Onanisme*. Lausanne: Marcuse Chapius et cie.

Wise, T. (1845). *Commentary on the Hindu System of Medicine*. Calcutta: Thacker.

Wolberg, L. (1948). *Medical Hypnosis*. New York: Grune and Stratton.

Wong, K., and Wu, L. (1936). *History of Chinese Medicine*. Shanghai: National Quarantine Service.

Yap, P. (1965). Koro: A culture-bound depersonalization syndrome. *British Journal of Psychiatry, 111*, 43–50.

CHAPTER 7

Alcohol and Erectile Failure

GORM WAGNER AND SØREN BUUS JENSEN

The effect of alcohol on sexual function will be discussed in two main sections. The first covers the effect of alcohol on normal sexual function. The other discusses sexual function in alcoholics. Some overlap, of course, is caused by the badly defined borderland between "normal" alcohol consumption and alcohol addiction.

Alcohol in Common Male Sexual Function

Alcohol is a centrally acting substance, which through the ages has been reputed to be an aphrodisiac. Alcohol acts as a general brain depressant and as a depressant on sexual performance, but the effect varies with the blood-alcohol concentration. In small doses, alcohol reduces anxiety and inhibitions, and social as well as sexual contact is made easier. In larger doses, it affects cognitive functions and further drinking may influence the state of consciousness similarly, to sedative drugs (Kaplan, 1974). Small doses of alcohol seem to increase libido, but in larger doses, the performance, although not the motivation, seems to be reduced in accordance with the classic words of Shakespeare: "[It] provokes the desire, but it takes away the performance" (Macbeth, Act II, Scene 3).

In younger males 26–45 years of age, without sexual dysfunction, alcohol is reported to influence ejaculation, causing ejaculation without pleasure, dry ejaculation, retarded ejaculation, and premature ejaculation (Jensen, 1979).

Only one experimental work has been published on the effect of acute alcohol intake on human erection (Farkas and Rosen, 1976). These authors gave alcohol in an amount unknown to the experimental subjects and aimed at blood-alcohol concentrations of 0.025%, 0.05%, and 0.07%, determined by breath analysis. The rate of penile tumescence measured by a circular strain gauge declined slightly at the lowest levels but more at 0.075%. Maximum tumescence was depressed at the larger doses as well. As only visual sexual stimulation was applied, the study shows only that penile tumescence response to that specific stimulus is reduced, not whether reflexogenic erection via the sacral cord is influenced.

The effect of acute alcohol intake on hormonal factors has been evaluated in some studies. At high blood levels, alcohol seems to suppress plasma testosterone; there is also a subsequent increase in plasma luteinizing hormone (LH) indicating that alcohol intake affects the pituitary–gonadal axis in normal males (Mendelson *et al.,* 1977). The sexual implications of such findings are unknown, but the demonstration of a correlation between plasma LH increase and sexual arousal may give new insights (Laferla *et al.,* 1976).

Alcoholism and Sexual Function

The difficulty of defining *alcoholism* generates insecurity about studies concerning sexual dysfunction and alcoholism. The haziness of the borderline between "normal drinking" and alcohol addiction is notorious. According to recent surveys, the alcoholic *dependence syndrome,* which is characterized by morning drinking, the critical point of no return, the physical symptoms of abstinence, and daily alcohol intake, seems to be the best way to distinguish alcoholics from nonalcoholics (Royal College of Psychiatrists, 1979).

Most studies concerning alcoholics' sexual function should be ignored because the methods and the definitions used and the descriptions of the patients included are not made specific enough. Furthermore, the sex partners of alcoholics are rarely evaluated. Most studies seem to be consistent in some data and rather inconsistent in others: while radioimmunoassays are described in the smallest detail, data on sexual functioning are often reported without any explanation of how they were collected. Furthermore, most studies are retrospective and uncontrolled. Studies of alcoholics including newer sexologic physiological methods are nearly absent (Jensen, 1978). Our knowledge concerning sexual function in alcoholic males is fragmentary and the following sections should be regarded as supplying only a few of the many pieces of a mosaic.

Sexual Life in Male Alcoholics

Alcoholics have in their histories an earlier sexual debut compared to nonalcoholics. Neither an early alcoholism debut nor an early sexual debut seems to be correlated with development of sexual dysfunction (Jensen, 1979).

Most alcoholics seem to have functioned well sexually for some years. Once the alcoholic condition progresses into the dependence syndrome and the drinking pattern becomes more uniform, the signs and symptoms of heavy drinking—be they social, psychiatric, or somatic—become more pronounced.

The alcoholic marriage has many problems. Studies by Burton and Kaplan

(1968) have shown the same frequency of sexual disturbances among alcoholics as among a matched group of partners in nonalcoholic marriages, although the symptoms were different. The alcoholic marriages were characterized by the husband's desire for higher sexual activity while the wife used denial of sex with an inebriated partner as a way of reducing the husband's alcohol intake. Many wives directly expressed their disgust with sexuality combined with alcohol intake. Student and Mantova (1969) showed that 35 out of the 40 wives of alcoholics studied experienced psychical disturbances, mostly of a depressive nature. This interactional phenomenon has been described in transaction-analytical terms by Steiner (1971) in *Games Alcoholics Play*. The wife often plays the role of "Persecutor" as well as "Rescuer." Such an analysis makes it clear that the counselor or therapist should be very much aware of "the function of the [sexual] dysfunction."

Sexual Dysfunction in Male Alcoholics

Frequencies of sexual disturbance in alcoholic men seem to vary from 8% (Lemere and Smith, 1973) to 63% (Jensen, 1979). This marked discrepancy illustrates the significance of the differences in methodology mentioned earlier.

Jensen (1979) found that 28% of addictive alcoholic males 30–40 years of age reported erectile failure. Reduced libido according to the subject's own expectation was mentioned by 36%, and 10% reported premature ejaculation. Retarded ejaculation, which has been previously described as a possible side effect of treatment with Antabuse® (disulfiram) (Martensen-Larsen, 1953) was seen in 16%. Among the many factors studied, erectile dysfunction was found particularly in men aged 40 or older, especially if they were single. The duration of alcoholism was not significantly related to sexual problems.

Alcohol and Sexual Function among Alcoholic Males

Nearly half of the sample of alcoholics in the study by Jensen (1979) reported sexual stimulation by alcohol intake, although many confirmed Shakespeare's postulate. In this same sample, 80% claimed that their partners would prefer sexual intercourse with a sober man. The remaining 20% said that they were always drunk at intercourse, and, among these, a higher frequency of sexual dysfunction was reported.

As for the etiology of sexual dysfunction in alcoholics, methodological problems, combined with the possibility of multifactorial influences, preclude a definite explanation. The theories are many, including neurological, hormonal, pharmacological, and psychosocial.

Neurological Factors. Alcoholic polyneuropathy is a well-known complication in chronic alcoholics, mainly affecting the somatic peripheral nerves. Disturbances of erection as well as of ejaculation are to be expected. Studies of reflexes, such as the bulbocavernosus reflex, have shown these to be often affected.

In a retrospective evaluation by Lemere and Smith (1973), neurological factors were considered of major significance, as sexual function was not restored after a year of sobriety. These factors are not at present well-elucidated and should be studied under well-defined conditions.

A factor often undetermined in such studies is alcoholic dementia. Recent studies (e.g., Lee *et al.,* 1979) examining alcoholics by CAT (computer axial tomography)-scanning and psychometric evaluation indicate a high rate of dementia, even in alcoholic males younger than 35. The consequences of such findings in relation to the personality structure of the alcoholic are obvious.

Hormonal Factors. As many as 80% of chronic alcoholics may experience decreased sex drive or impotence (Van Thiel and Lester, 1976). Up to 80% may also show signs of testicular atrophy. Abnormalities in estrogen secretion or metabolism may be responsible for the gynecomastia seen in 20% (Van Thiel and Lester, 1979).

There is increasing evidence that alcohol has a direct toxic effect on the testes as well as on the hypothalamic–pituitary system. In normal volunteers, testosterone fell to 20% of control values 12–20 hr after the ingestion of sufficient alcohol to produce a moderate to severe hangover (Ylikahri *et al.,* 1974). Also in normals, the frequency and amplitude of gonadotropin secretory bursts is decreased after alcohol consumption (Gordon and Southern, 1977). When alcohol consumption is continual over 72 hr, gonadotropins no longer respond to lowered levels of testosterone (Van Thiel *et al.,* 1978).

Chronic alcoholics typically do not show normal elevations of follicle-stimulating hormone (FSH) and LH in response to clomiphene (Van Thiel *et al.,* 1974), and LH responses to LH-RH (releasing hormone) are also inadequate (Van Thiel *et al.,* 1978).

Another hormone frequently elevated in alcoholics is prolactin (Lindholm *et al.,* 1978a,b; Panerai *et al.,* 1977). Prolactin may modulate the level of estrogen receptors in liver (Chamners *et al.,* 1975) and LH receptors in testes (Zipf and Payne, 1977).

While there is clinical evidence of high estrogenic action in alcoholics, free estradiol levels are usually normal (Kley *et al.,* 1979), although plasma estrone may be elevated (Kley *et al.,* 1975). It has been suggested that there is increased steroid aromatization to estrogen within tissues because the steroids bypass the diseased liver (Van Thiel and Lester, 1979). Other evidence from the rat suggests that a decrease in testosterone results in an increase in estrogen receptors in the liver (Eagon *et al.,* 1978).

Thus, the role of estrogen, as well as of other hormones, in the changes in sexual behavior reported by alcoholics must be more fully elucidated.

Pharmacological Factors. Antabuse® (disulfiram) is commonly used in alcoholism treatment. The drug has some reputation as an impotence-inducing factor. This claim, well-known to all alcoholic treatment teams, is repudiated by recent studies. The study of Jensen (1979) showed that most alcoholic males experienced sexual dysfunction from their first day of Antabuse® but reported the same frequency of sexual activity (intercourse as well as masturbation) during the month before and after this first treatment day. This finding indicates a shift in the qualitative experience of sexuality without any quantitative change. Martensen-Larsen (1953) reported retarded ejaculation as a possible side effect of Antabuse® treatment, but this symptom was relatively infrequent among the sexual disturbances reported in the study of Jensen.

A recent (and astonishing) study by Kristensen (1973) revealed, in a double-blind crossover study of the side effects of Antabuse®, a significantly higher rate of sexual disturbances in the *placebo* group.

The claims against Antabuse® should be seen as part of the ambivalence of beginning the treatment for alcoholism. Furthermore, a change from daily heavy drinking to alcohol abstinence, and possibly the minor tranquilizing drugs given for the physical abstinence symptoms, seems a reasonable explanation for the qualitative changes reported.

Psychosocial Factors. These aspects are many; some have already been touched on. Ambivalence about treatment, the changing power-balance at home, the personality structure of the patient and the partner as well as their interactions, existence as a chronic diseased person with daily restrictions in social life, poor self-esteem, and social deprivations—all are possible factors. In the community and outside of marriage exist a relatively large group of single, middle-aged men with low social esteem and problems with establishing long-standing relationships. The problems of these people may have caused the impression of reduced heterosexual interest in alcoholic males (Levine, 1955) as well as conjectures on the relationship of alcoholism and homosexuality (Machover *et al.*, 1959). The study of Jensen (1979) showed no overrepresentation of homosexuals among alcoholic males (3%).

Treatment of Sexual Dysfunction in Alcoholic Males

A specific medical history combined with objective measures should be the basis of any consultation. As a common rule, it should be emphasized to the alcoholic patient that alcohol abuse should be stopped before any kind of sex therapy is instituted. Some months of sobriety should be required, even though some alcoholics claim to drink because of their sexual problems. A fear of additional sexual problems caused by Antabuse® seems not to be justified as an excuse for deferring alcoholism treatment. The vicious circle has to be stopped somewhere. Even if the alcoholic should declare that alcohol by itself is not the main problem, neither is sexual dysfunction.

The psychosocial factors described above should be well elucidated in each case, along with possible somatic influences. In a great number of alcoholics, some underlying somatic problems may also be related to the etiology of sexual disturbances. It should be remembered that an organic factor is often followed by a superimposed psychogenic symptom pattern. The symptom, by itself, rarely gives the explicit etiological diagnosis.

Complaints of Antabuse®-induced sexual dysfunction should be used as an invitation to discuss the interactional problems with patient and partner, rather than as an excuse for discontinuing Antabuse®. The psychopharmacological treatment should be carefully chosen; nonaddictive drugs that have low interference with sexual function should be used. In patients demonstrating signs of polyneuropathy, a B-vitamin regimen might be indicated. Selected cases may be referred to sexological treatment. Specific diagnostic procedures are discussed in Chapter 8.

Conclusion

Sexual dysfunctions are common in alcoholics. Alcohol affects both the body (CNS and peripheral nerves) and the interpersonal relationships of the alcoholic. Thus, it is of great importance to evaluate the patient's total situation. It seems most likely that Antabuse® *per se* does not cause erectile dysfunction. It should be stressed that the alcoholism should be treated before, or at least concomitantly with, sex therapy.

References

Burton, G., and Kaplan, H. M. (1968). Sexual behaviour and adjustment of married alcoholics. *Quarterly Journal of Studies of Alcohol, 29*, 603–609.

Chamners, G., Costolow, M., and McGuire, W. (1975). Estrogen receptor in rat liver and its dependence on prolactin. *Steroids, 26*, 363–371.

Eagon, P., Imhoff, A., and Fisher, S. (1978). Estrogen receptors of male and female liver. *Clinical Research, 26*, 317A.

Farkas, G. M., and Rosen, R. C. (1976). Effect of alcohol on elicited male sexual response. *Journal of Studies on Alcohol, 37*, 265–272.

Gordon, G., and Southern, A. (1977). Metabolic effects of alcohol on the endocrine system. In C. S. Lieber (Ed.), *Metabolic Aspects of Alcoholism*. Baltimore: University Park Press.

Jensen, S. B. (1978). *Sexual Dysfunction and Diabetes Mellitus*. Gold Medal Project in Medicine, University of Copenhagen.

Jensen, S. B. (1979). Sexual customs and sexual dysfunction in alcoholics. *British Journal of Sexual Medicine, 53*, 29–30, and *54*, 30–34.

Jensen, S. B. (1980). Sexual dysfunction in general practice. *Ugeskrift for Laeger*, Copenhagen.

Kaplan, H. S. (1974). *The New Sex Therapy*. London: Bailliere and Tindall.

Kley, H., Niesclag, E., Wiegelman, W., Solback, H., and Kruskemper, M. (1975). Steroid hormones and their binding in plasma of male patients with fatty liver, chronic hepatitis, and liver cirrhosis. *Acta Endocrinologia, 79*, 275–285.

Kley, H., Storkmeyer, G., and Kruskemper, H. (1979). Effect of testosterone application on hormone concentration of androgens and estrogen in male patients with cirrhosis of the liver. *Gastroenterology, 76*, 235–241.

Kristensen, J. K. (1973). Side-effects in disulfiram-treatment. *Ugeskrift for Laeger,* Copenhagen *135*, 1457–1459.

Laferla, J. J., Andersson, D. L., and Schalach, D. S. (1976). Psychoendocrine response to visual erotic stimulation in human males. *Psychosomatic Medicine, 38*, 62.

Lee, K., Hardt, F., Moller, L., Haubek, A., and Jensen, E. (1979). Alcohol induced brain damage and liver damage in young males. *The Lancet, I*, 759–761.

Lemere, F., and Smith, J. W. (1973). Alcohol induced sexual impotence. *American Journal of Psychiatry, 130*, 212–213.

Levine, J. (1955). The sexual adjustment of alcoholics. *Quarterly Journal of Studies of Alcohol, 16*, 675–680.

Lindholm, J., Fabricius-Bjerre, N., Bahnsen, M., Boiesen, P., Bangstrup, L., Pedersen, M. L., and Hagen, C. (1978a). Pituitary–testicular function in patients with chronic alcoholism. *European Journal of Clinical Investigation, 8*, 269–272.

Lindholm, J., Fabricius-Bjerre, N., Bahnsen, M., Boiesen, P., Hagen, C., and Christensen, T. (1978b). Sex steroids and sex-hormone binding globulin in males with chronic alcoholism. *European Journal of Clinical Investigation, 8*, 273–276.

Machover, S., Puzzo, F. S., Machover, K., and Plumeau, F. (1959). Clinical and objective studies of personality variables in alcoholics. III. An objective study of homosexuality in alcoholism. *Quarterly Journal of Studies of Alcohol, 20*, 528–542.

Martensen-Larsen, I. (1953). Five years experience with disulfiram (Antabuse) in the treatment of alcoholics. *Quarterly Journal of Studies of Alcohol, 14*, 406–418.

Mendelson, J. H., Mello, N. K., and Ellingboe, J. (1977). Effects of acute alcohol intake on pituitary–gonadal hormones in normal human males. *The Journal of Pharmacology and Experimental Therapeutics, 202*, 676–682.

Panerai, A., Salerno, F., Manneschi, M., *et al.* (1977). Growth hormone and prolactin responses to thyrotropin releasing hormone in patients with severe liver disease. *Journal of Clinical Endocrinology and Metabolism, 45*, 134–140.

The Royal College of Psychiatrists. (1979). *Alcohol and Alcoholism.* London: Tavistock Publications.

Steiner, C. (1971). *Games Alcoholics Play.* New York: Grove Press.

Student, V., and Mantova, A. (1969). Development of mental disorders in wives of alcoholics. *Czechoslovakian Psychiatrie, 65*, 23–29.

Van Thiel, D., and Lester, R. (1976). Sex and alcohol: A second peak. *New England Journal of Medicine, 295*, 835–836.

Van Thiel, D., and Lester, R. (1979). The effect of chronic alcohol abuse on sexual function. *Clinics in Endocrinology and Metabolism, 8*, 499–510.

Van Thiel, D., Lester, D., and Sherins, R. (1974). Hypogonadism in alcoholic liver disease: evidence for a double defect. *Gastroenterology, 67*, 1188–1199.

Van Thiel, D., Lester, D., and Vaitukaitis, T. (1978). Evidence for a defect in pituitary secretion of luteinizing hormone in chronic alcoholic men. *Journal of Clinical Endocrinology, 47*, 499–507.

Ylikahri, R., Huttunen, M., and Harkonen, M., *et al.* (1974). Low plasma testosterone values in men during hangover. *Journal of Steroid Biochemistry, 5*, 655–658.

Zipf, W., and Payne, A. (1977). Modulation of LH receptors by luteinizing hormone, prolactin, and growth hormone. Abstract submitted to 59th Annual Meeting of the Endocrine Society.

CHAPTER 8

Methods for Differential Diagnosis of Psychogenic and Organic Erectile Failure

GORM WAGNER

Diagnostic Approach to the Patient with Erectile Failure

It is a general belief that an increasing number of impotent patients have sought out doctors during the last 5–10 years. It is documented that the medical profession generally has had very little education in sexual medicine, so that patients are highly dependent on the specific physician contacted. Therefore, one of the aims of this book is to outline possible diagnostic approaches. While in the clinical situation the doctor's first impression of the patient is important, it is crucial that this first impression not mislead the doctor into believing that the problem is or is not psychogenic. The postulated ratio of psychogenic to organic dysfunction varies from 20:1 to 1:7. In the future, the examination of patients by means of new and more sophisticated diagnostic procedures may tell us the true proportion. However, this ratio may vary from one cultural area to the next, depending on the given society, its social structure, and its religious ethic. Also, sexological clinics in association with psychiatric departments or psychological institutions may receive another type of patient than the internist, the urologist, the andrologist, or the vascular surgeon. Characteristic of the group of males complaining of erectile dysfunction is heterogeneity. It should be kept in mind that failure of erection is a symptom that can have a variety of etiologies and that the diagnostic procedure for finding the correct etiology may be rather cumbersome. The family physician who is well educated in sexual medicine and is aware of the many possibilities that may cause erectile dysfunction should, with basic knowledge of the patient, be in the best position to manage the evaluation.

Table VII outlines a format for a plan of medical examination of the man with erectile problems. Information should be conveyed to the patient at the earliest occasion. In some clinics, material is sent to the patient along with a questionnaire that the patient is asked to fill in or to bring to first consultation. Barry and Hodges (1978) advocated sending a questionnaire to the patient when he was referred to a specialist's office and asking him to return it before the first consultation. This procedure forces the patient to think about his situation and may make him realize for the first time that he has to experience a series of investigations and consultations. This approach discourages some men from continuing with evaluation and thereby helps to select highly motivated patients.

Of primary importance in the history is obtaining a precise description of the dysfunction to ascertain that the complaint is not based on premature ejaculation. Recently, a more systematic approach has been suggested to create a scientific nosology within the area of erectile failure (Graber, 1979). In a two-year review of all men in a sexual therapy clinic, Graber evaluated 468 men, of whom 34% were normal partners of a female seeking help, 34% were men with erectile failure, and the rest were men with ejaculatory disorders.

Table VII. Plan of Medical Examination of the Dysfunctional Man[a]

General:	
History	
Information to patient	
Physical status (including vascular status)	
Neurological examination	
Blood tests (hormones, sugar, creatinine)	
Noninvasive, "specific":	
Genital reflexes	
(Cystometry)	
Stimulation plethysmography	visual vibration
Penile blood pressure	rest postocclusive
Penile pulse amplitude (Doppler)	rest postocclusive
Nocturnal plethysmography (NPT)	laboratory home
Invasive, specific:	
Blood flow (xenon washout)	rest stimulation postocclusive
Passive erection (by infusion)	
Infusion cavernosography	rest stimulation
Arteriography	

[a]From Wagner (1979).

Table VIII. Subtypes of Erectile Failure in Relation to Function[a]

Subtype	Criteria
Erectile failure with intercourse, primary/always	A male who has never been functional in intercourse because of a continuous history of erectile failure.
Erectile failure with intercourse, primary/sometimes	Although the male has generally had a history of erectile failure with intercourse, he is occasionally functional. However, he is never free of anxiety regarding his dysfunction.
Erectile failure with intercourse, secondary/always	A male who was formerly functional but is now dysfunctional all of the time in intercourse because of erectile failure.
Erectile failure with intercourse, secondary/sometimes	A male who was formerly functional but is now dysfunctional in intercourse some of the time because of erectile failure.

[a]Modified from Graber (1979).

The first task is to subdivide the patients with erectile failure into primary and secondary cases. Graber further subdivides according to whether the dysfunction was always or sometimes present (Table VIII). In Table IX, the 157 men in Graber's study are listed according to this subdivision, and the relative incidences are shown. In the sample, about 20% of the cases were primary cases.

The duration, development, and degree of the erectile dysfunction should be thoroughly elucidated, including rigidity and morning erections, and whether the failure exists in all intercourse positions and with different partners. Quite often a man who starts having difficulties with erection tries to see whether he is able to erect with another woman. Medication, alcohol consumption, and smoking habits should be evaluated. Only occasionally is it possible to make a certain diagnosis from the history alone, and a plan for examinations should be made. These may follow the suggestions in Table VII. The individual examinations are discussed in the following paragraphs.

Sexual Stimulation

Few clinics apply this procedure, which is a logical one in that it is the ability to erect in connection with sexual arousal that is problematic. Figure 26 demonstrates six patients exposed to the same visual sexual stimulation consisting of a taped series of nine sequences, each of 150-sec duration. Film has been found to elicit a significantly better response than slides (Bancroft, 1976) and should be shown for no less than 120 sec. The series have been selected from commercially available pornographic films and have been selected for content in order to provide

Table IX. Coital Erectile Failure[a]

	N			% Total of erectile failure cases		
Primary always						
Unknown erection	0			0		
Full erection	4			2.5		
Partial erection	3			1.9		
Full and partial erection	5			3.2		
	12			7.6		
Primary sometimes						
Unknown erection	1			.6		
Full erection	5			3.2		
Partial erection	8			5.1		
Full and partial erection	5			3.2		
	19			12.1		
		31			19.7	
Secondary always						
Unknown erection	1			.6		
Full erection	6			3.8		
Partial erection	19			12.1		
Full and partial erection	4			2.5		
	30			19.0		
Secondary sometimes						
Unknown erection	7			4.5		
Full erection	30			19.1		
Partial erection	26			16.6		
Full and partial erection	33			21.0		
	96			61.2		
		126			80.2	
			157			100

[a]Modified from Graber (1979).

the greatest diversity. The patient is seated in a chair in a quiet room, preferably noise-reduced, and is given an explanation of what is going to occur. He is also asked to concentrate on the film and if possible to add fantasy. The strain gauge is placed around the shaft of the penis.

All positive responses are of value as they may indicate the speed of tumescence and may show which sequence gives the best response. This latter information may be used later when other measurements are taken. Repeated exposures to the same stimuli may cause methodological problems: either they may reduce inhibition, thus increasing penile response, or they may be habituating, thus reducing penile response. A negative response is not explainable because of limited experience with such materials. The curve with no response in Figure 26A was from a man with psychogenic erectile dysfunction.

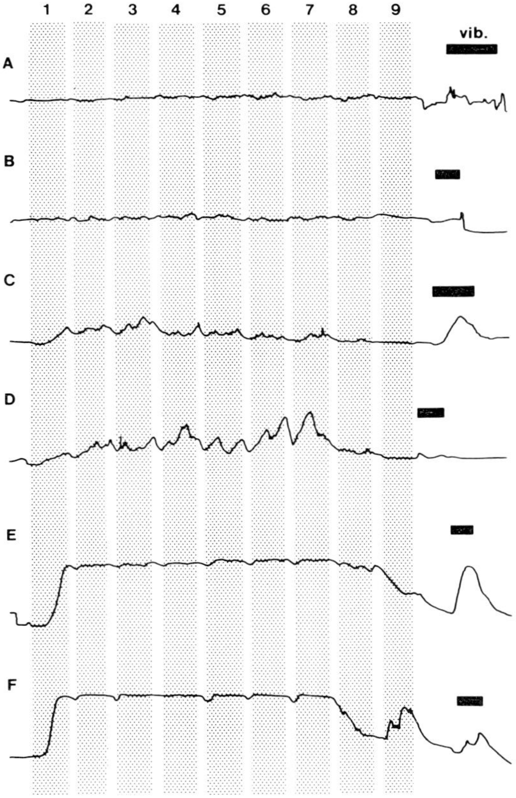

Figure 26. Curves from circumferential strain-gauge measurements in six men complaining of erectile dysfunction exposed to visual sexual stimulation (VSS). Numbers 1–9 indicate periods of VSS (erotic filmstrips), each of 150-sec duration with different content, Number 9 showing male homosexual activity. The horizontal black bar indicates a period of direct penile vibration (vib) with a frequency changing from 40 to 80 Hz. A: 62-year-old with secondary erectile dysfunction (sec.e.d.), with almost no reaction to VSS and an uncertain response to vib. Diagnosed as psychogenic. B: 42-year-old primary erectile dysfunction (prim.e.d.), bisexual. Diagnosed as possibly psychogenic. C: 72-year-old sec.e.d., slow and modest filling during VSS, positive but slow vib response. Arterial insufficiency. D: 24-year-old prim.e.d. Slow tumescence and low filling during VSS, no reaction to vib. Bilateral arterial dysplasia. E: 40-year-old sec.e.d. Response to VSS and vib normal. No abnormal findings in other tests or psychological evaluation. Undiagnosed. F: 22-year-old prim.e.d. Maximal and fast response to VSS. Some reaction to Sequence 9. Slight vib reaction, abnormal venous drainage.

It is obvious that the clinical situation may produce distracting thoughts and emotions that may influence the response, but it is an unanswered question whether a man vulnerable to such a situation is also more likely to be disturbed in his home situation. The necessity of visual stimulation during the penile blood-flow measurement and infusion cavernosography will be discussed later. Kolářský and Madlafousek (1977) studied the serial effect in phallometric experiments in 56 young men. It was found that any stimulus with which the experiment started had a weaker effect than when it was presented later in the series, and also that the response to a given stimulus was influenced by the preceding stimulus. No habituation effect was found. No such studies have been performed in older age groups. Sexual stimulation in the laboratory setting is a valuable tool in research (Geer, 1976) and most probably also in clinical diagnostic procedures, although its precise role remains to be defined.

Morning Erections

The phenomenon of morning erection (erection at the time of wakening) has been the subject of only a few studies. Karacan (1970) studied 10 normal men in a sleep laboratory. Of these subjects, 5 were awakened two hours before their usual time and asked to urinate and defecate. They then returned to sleep. The other 5 slept without interruption. No difference in the erection on awakening at the normal time could be noticed in the two groups. This experiment suggests that morning erection is not due to bladder distension. The significance of changes in morning erection patterns in normal men and in men with erectile failure remains obscure.

Genital Reflexes

As peripheral nerves may be involved in erectile failure it is necessary to evaluate genital reflexes in addition to a general neurological examination and the more special tests mentioned in Chapter 5, such as the beat-to-beat variation during evaluation of autonomic function.

The cremasteric reflex is ipsilateral, superficial, and somatic. It is elicited by stroking the skin of the inner side of the thigh with a blunt point. The response consists of elevation of the ipsilateral testicle. The reflex is mediated by the ileoinguinal and genitofemoral nerves, with centers in the first and second lumbar segments. The evoked contraction of the cremasteric muscle is slow and resembles that seen during sexual arousal with erection (Wagner, 1976). Absence of the reflex may be due to lesions in any part of the peripheral reflex arc as well as in the central motor neuron.

The scrotal reflex is axonal and local. It is often noticed in a man who undresses in a cold room. The response is a slow vermicular contraction of the dartos muscle, elicited by application of a cold object to the scrotum, the perineum, or the upper inner part of the thigh. It may be absent in patients with myelopathies.

The bulbocavernosus reflex is bilateral, spinal, and somatic. The reflex arc runs afferently and efferently through the pudendal nerve, with the reflex center in the second and third sacral cord segment. By pinching the dorsum of the glans or applying gentle pressure to the glans, the reflex is elicited. The response consists of a contraction of the bulbocavernous muscle and the external anal sphincter. The reflex can also be quantified by electrical stimulation (Figure 27) applied by a ring electrode around the glans and an EMG recording by an electrode inserted in the bulbocavernous muscle (Vacek and Lachman, 1977). In normal, potent men, a mean reflex latency time of 35 ± 1.2 msec was found, while a group of 20 diabetics suffering from erectile dysfunction exhibited a prolonged latency period (45.8 ± 4.3 msec). It should be noted, as by Blaivas *et al.* (1980), that prolongation of the latency period does not indicate a direct cause-and-effect relationship to erectile failure. In their study of 27 men referred for erectile impotence, they found that almost half of the men had combinations of neurological, psychological, and vascular abnormal findings.

The superficial anal reflex is bilateral, somatic, and superficial, with the center in the second, third, and fourth sacral segments. When the skin of the perineal region is stroked, a contraction of the external anal sphincter is seen.

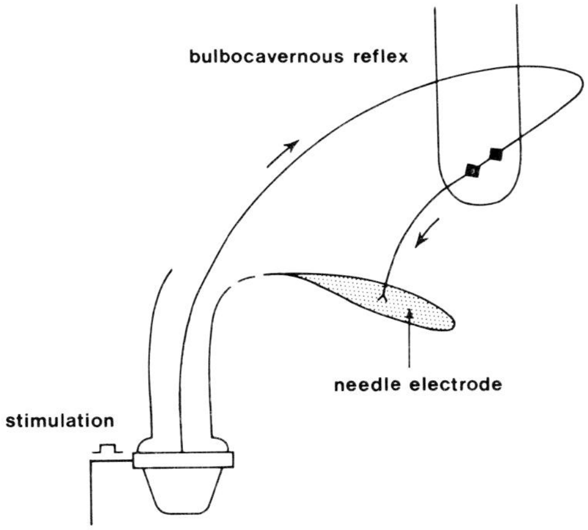

Figure 27. Recording of the bulbocavernous reflex. Schematic drawing of ring electrode, reflex arc, and EMG recording. (After Vacek and Lachman, 1977.)

The internal anal reflex may be used for the evaluation of the sympathetic elements of the hypogastric nerve and the presacral plexus, with a presumed center in the first and second lumbar segments. The reflex is elicited by introducing a gloved finger into the anus and consists of contraction of the internal anal sphincter.

The value of these examinations in the daily clinical evaluation of erectile dysfunction is not known. But the existence of the reflexes gives an assurance of the normal neurological status in that region. Still better and somewhat more logical would be to examine the erection itself, provoked by reflex. One way of producing a reflexogenic erection is via local vibration.

Vibration Tests

Vibration sensitivity decreases with aging, especially after age 40 (Steiness, 1957), and also in relation to peripheral neuropathy in diabetics (Jersild and Lauritzen, 1957). Also, a more generalized decrease in tactile sensitivity occurs with aging (Weiss, 1971), along with an increase in the average threshold to vibration of the penis (Newman, 1970).

Thresholds can vary in relation to location and sexual function. Thresholds at the corona of 100 males with no urological or sexual complaints were found to be lower than those at the tip of the glans in 65%, the same in 20%, and higher in 15% (Newman, 1970). In 56 healthy married men, penile sensitivity and the frequency of intercourse were compared. A close correlation was found.

For clinical purposes, a vibrator with a frequency of 60 Hz can be applied to the frenulum of the penis, and the threshold for perception can be expressed in volts (Biothesiometer), as described by Lundberg (1978). Unfortunately, there seem to be no published data as to the validity of the test as a diagnostic tool in erectile dysfunction.

In the study by Edwards and Husted (1976) of 18 normal men, the vibrotactile threshold was measured at the tip of the finger, at the toe, and at the frenulum of the flaccid and erect penis. Expressed in decibels (db), the mean threshold to vibration was finger (37 db), toe (50.9 db), flaccid penis (45.8 db), and erect penis (53 db). The difference between erection and flaccidity is significant and might be explained by a "thinning out" of the receptors under the probe with the tissue stretched. An experiment like this is, however, difficult to perform, as environmental influences may affect the subject concurrently with the erotic stimulation.

A more direct approach would be to evaluate the result of penile vibration, that is, erection (and/or ejaculation). Some spermatologists make use of a vibrator to collect semen for examination. An apparatus that can be used for such studies

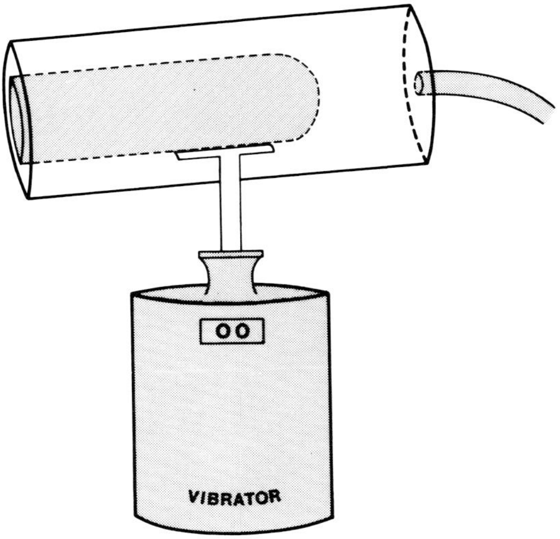

Figure 28. Vibrophalloplethysmograph, originally designed by G. S. Brindley, London, and modified and described by Wagner and Brindley (1980). For description see text.

is shown in Figure 28. It is designed as a combined vibrophalloplethysmograph, which makes it possible to study the change in volume and circumference when a circular strain gauge is placed around the penis (Wagner and Brindley, 1980). The penis is covered with a condom and placed in the tube, which is made airtight by folding the condom around the collar. Connection via a large volume bottle is made to a pressure transducer as in ordinary volume plethysmography, and the calibration is performed. The plate on which the penis is placed is connected to a vibrator by a movable rod that can be regulated by remote control to give variable frequency and amplitude. The problem is that not all normal experimental subjects respond to vibration. Thus, in a case with a negative result, the vibration test has limited clinical value. Furthermore, a given male who once responds to vibration will continue to do so at repeated visits to the laboratory. A frequency between 40 and 80 Hz seems to be optimal in most cases. In some cases, a change of frequency seems most effective. A negative respondent has never shown a positive response later, although he might experience erection from visual sexual stimulation in experimental sessions at a time when he has accommodated to the situation. Figure 29 demonstrates a set of recordings obtained from strain gauge and volume plethysmography simultaneously in a young male who responded well to vibration. We have found that for clinical purposes, it is not necessary to record the volume changes, as they are highly related to strain gauge measurements, a method of more technical simplicity.

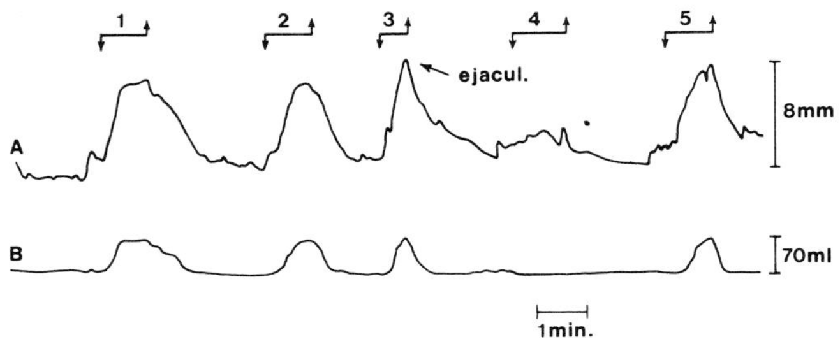

Figure 29. Two original recordings made simultaneously of (A) circumference of the penis by mercury strain gauge and (B) change of volume during erection. During Periods 1–5 vibration to the penis was applied by remote control. At the third vibration (3), the man ejaculated, and the vibration was interrupted. After two minutes, another vibration period was initiated (4), but no erection was provoked as he was still in the refractory period. At Period 5, he was responding again, but with slower tumescence than before. The good concordance between circumference and volume change should be noted.

Conclusion

The determination of vibration sensitivity may be of some additional help as can be a positive erectile response to vibration in diagnosing the cause of dysfunction. Additional studies of these methods in dysfunctional males are much needed.

Cystometry

The principle of cystometry is the recording of variations of pressure in the bladder at various degrees of filling (pressure/volume curve). The shape of the obtained curve yields information about tonus and possible inclination to spasticity. Also, the method can give information regarding voiding pressure. As it is necessary to do catheterization via the urethra, the amount of residual urine can also be determined.

Since the detrusor muscle and the smooth muscles involved in erection are innervated from the same sacral roots and are presumably closely interconnected, it has been suggested that a neurogenic dysfunction of the bladder would be an indication of a similar condition of the nervous control of erection. In a single case of diabetes mellitus, Barry and Hodges (1978) found a large bladder (750 ml) and 180 ml of residual urine. No other information on neurological objective findings was given. Ellenberg (1971) examined 71 diabetics and found that 90% of the 41 dysfunctional as against 10% of the 30 functional men exhibited a neurogenic bladder. Whether other neurological examinations would yield the same indication of a neurogenic erectile dysfunction is not known. One should observe, however, that the procedure of catheterization entails some hazards and that there may be pain for some days after the examination. Until more studies are presented on the value of this examination as a differential diagnostic procedure in erectile dysfunction, it might be advisable not to use this method as a matter of routine.

Penile Blood-Pressure Measurement

The penile pulse can be felt by compressing each cavernous body between the thumb and the forefinger. This simple procedure may provide gross information on the arteries and the pressure within the vessels. In a palpation study of several hundred men, Canning *et al.* (1963) found diminished potency in all 31 men without a palpable pulse. The palpation of small arteries is, however, a dubious affair, and clinical experience with arteriography has told us not to rely on digital palpation.

A simple diagnostic noninvasive method for evaluation of the arterial supply is blood pressure measurement. Some investigators (Britt *et al.*, 1971; Gaskell, 1971) advocated this method as a diagnostic tool in vascular occlusive dysfunction at a time when no diagnostic methods were available for determination of penile blood flow. As the simple method of the mercury strain gauge had been described some years earlier, it seemed easy, using a small blood pressure cuff, to perform measurements on the penis. The gauge consists of a small-caliber silicone tube filled with mercury placed around the penis. The change of length due to change of circumference is recorded by measuring the change of resistance in the mercury column. Figure 30 shows schematically the arrangement used by most clinicians and indicates that the brachial blood pressure is measured simultaneously with

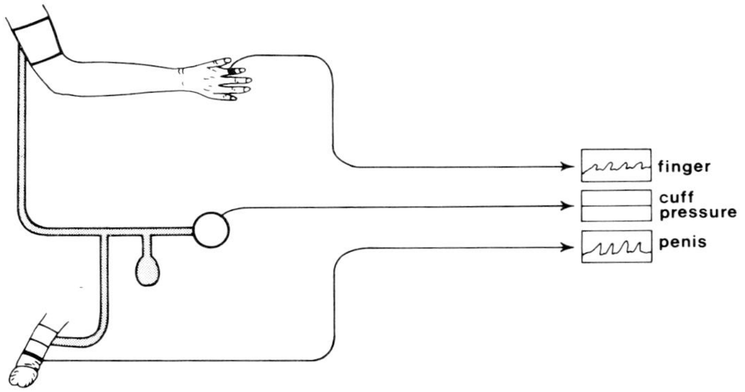

Figure 30. Schematic drawing of simultaneous blood-pressure measurement in arm and penis by application of circular strain gauges peripheral to the pneumatic cuffs. (Modified from Britt *et al.*, 1971.)

that of the penis. The examination takes place in a quiet room with the patient lying in a supine position. A baseline pulse curve is obtained from both measure points. Both pneumatic cuffs are inflated simultaneously above the systolic pressure. The pressure of the cuffs and the two pulse curves are recorded simultaneously. The pressure is then gradually taken off (preferably automatically) as shown in Figure 31. At a certain point, the pulse curve reappears for each of the two areas measured, and each pressure is noted.

Measurement of the postocclusive reactive hyperemia phase after 4 min of complete arterial closure was introduced by Britt *et al.* (1971). The ultrasound Doppler technique, applying an 8-MHz transducer recessed in the penile cuff, was introduced by Abelson (1975). This procedure makes it possible to evaluate the systolic as well as the diastolic level in the penile artery (Figure 32).

Examination of single penile arteries and evaluation of the occurrence and the appearance of the pulse-velocity curve has been used by some clinicians and correlated with findings from arteriography. Selective examinations of the two dorsal and the two deep arteries of the penis were done in 55 men with erectile

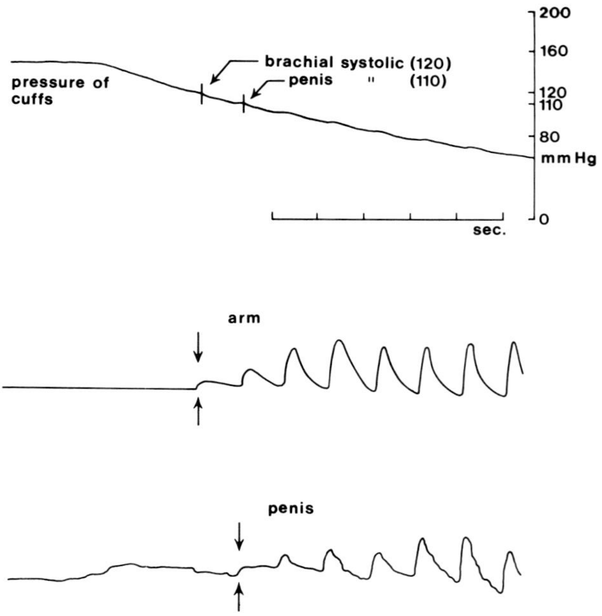

Figure 31. Simultaneous recording of pressure in cuffs of arm and penis and pulse amplitude at both sites. The pressure is slowly released and the systolic pressure noted in the arm and the penis. The PBPI (penile blood pressure index) is calculated. In this case, it is 110/120 = 0.91.

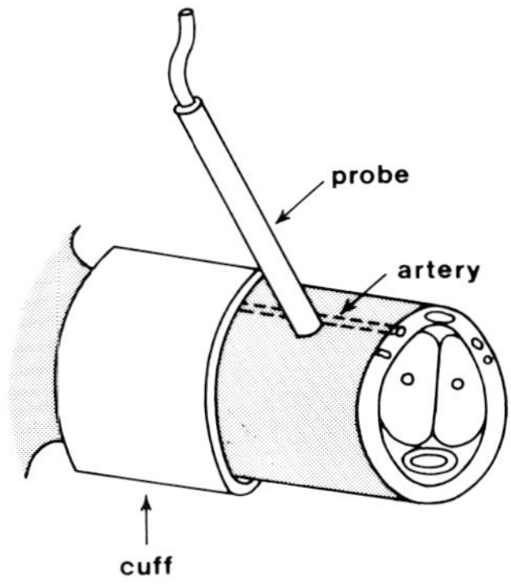

Figure 32. Schematic drawing of pneumatic cuff around the penis and the Doppler probe, which can also be recessed in the cuff.

dysfunction (Juhan *et al.,* 1978a). With the patient in the supine position, the dorsal arteries are located under the symphysis. When the penis is placed with the tip pointing toward the umbilicus, the deep arteries are located with the probe placed in the penoscrotal junction. Figure 33 demonstrates normal and abnormal pulse curves of dysfunctional patients. In 50 of 55 patients, abnormal Doppler findings were noted; of these 50 patients, 49 had demonstrable arterial lesions found at arteriography. Five normal Doppler curves were verified by five normal arteriograms. Also, in a study of 103 cases of erectile dysfunction, Virag (1980a)

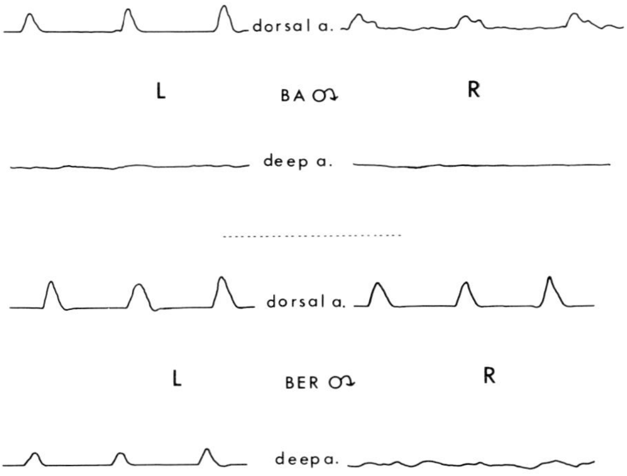

Figure 33. Doppler curves from single arteries in two men with erectile dysfunction. BA shows an abnormal configuration of the right dorsal penile artery and no detectable pulse in any of the deep penile arteries. BER shows an abnormal right deep artery. In both patients, arterial lesions were found by arteriography. (Courtesy of Dr. C. M. Juhan, Marseille.)

found a high correlation of positive Doppler findings with pathological arteriographic findings.

In order to provide more objective analysis of the Doppler findings, Velcek *et al.* (1980) have introduced "the penile flow index." This index is expressed by the average penile acceleration (peak velocity over pulse rise time) relative to the radial artery acceleration. The average penile acceleration is determined by the sum of the accelerations found in both deep arteries and one dorsal artery divided by 3. This method of calculation has led to better diagnosis of cases with arterial insufficiency.

Most authors make use of a *penile blood-pressure index* (PBPI) given as a penile systolic value divided by the brachial systolic value. Normals have been found to exhibit a systolic blood pressure in the penis similar to that in the arm, and a penile blood pressure of 20 mm Hg or more below the arm pressure is considered abnormal (Britt *et al.,* 1971). In 40 patients with a history of dysfunction, 10 were found with a considerably abnormal penis pulse curve and a decrease of blood pressure. In 2 patients who had aortoiliac occlusive disease and who had reconstructive arterial surgery, the penile plethysmography studies indicated improvement after surgery.

Abelson (1975) studied 29 normal subjects and 50 dysfunctional diabetics. By palpation, the arteries could be felt in all the normals but could not be recognized in 6 of the diabetics. The penile blood pressure was obtained in all the normals, but not in 2 of the diabetics. The author classified as normal a penile blood pressure as low as 50 mm Hg lower than the brachial systolic pressure. These findings were confirmed by Engel, Burnham, and Carter (1978), who found a mean index (PBPI) of 0.96 in a control group of normal men, whereas a mean of 0.59 was found in vascular impotence.

Another study describing a penile blood-pressure index is that of Gaylis (1978). He found 0.7 in a group of 40 patients with aortoiliac thrombosis, 5 of whom were dysfunctional. After surgery, 4 of the 5 regained function and the penile pressure index increased. He considered a pressure index of 0.8 critical and emphasized that one does not always find recurrence of potency after surgery, as the intervention may damage pelvic nerve plexuses and yet bring about normal arterial blood pressure in the flaccid penis.

It should be remembered that blood pressure measurement is always done on the flaccid penis and therefore tells only about the resting system. It does not give a picture of the functional state during the tumescent phase, although the appearance of the pulse amplitude may indicate pathology even without the pressure measurement (Figure 34).

Kempczinski (1979) examined 106 patients referred either for evaluation of intermittent claudication or for erectile dysfunction. In general, the sexually dysfunctional patients were older and had a much greater frequency of associated diseases than the sexually functional men. The PBPI was 0.99 in 9 functional

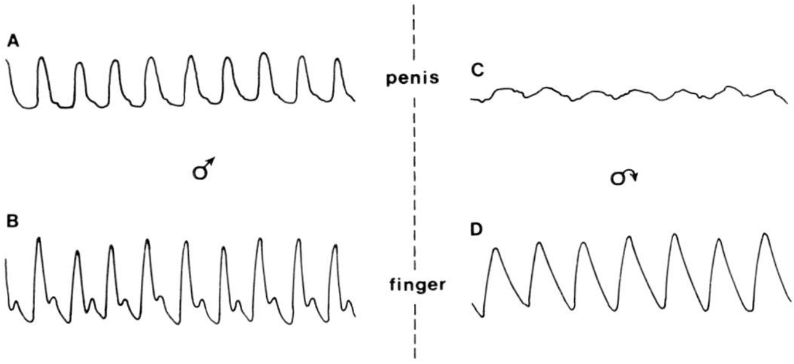

Figure 34. Pulse amplitude from penis and finger (A and B) in a functional man and (C and D) in a man with aortoiliac thrombosis and dysfunction.

patients below 40 years of age, but only 0.74 in 29 dysfunctional patients in same age group. In 5 men above 40, and functional, the PBPI was 0.84, while in the 64 men above 40 years, and dysfunctional, the PBPI was only 0.58. The author claimed that atherosclerotic narrowing of the pelvic vasculature with its resultant decrease in penile blood flow is an inevitable consequence of aging, and that in some patients with more advanced forms of the disease, it may cause dysfunction. A postischemic reactive hyperemia, as judged by an increase in pulse amplitude, was seen in all patients under 40 years. In 45 older patients, it was present in two-thirds, with no differences between functional and dysfunctional patients.

Recently, strain gauge plethysmography and the ultrasonic Doppler technique were simultaneously applied by Metz and Bengtsson (1980). They found by this double determination a coefficient of variation of 6.3% by repeated determinations in normal men. In patients with atherosclerotic disease in the legs, a penile blood pressure index lower than 0.6 was associated with dysfunction in more than 90% (Figure 25). When the positive and negative predictive values were compared, the false classifications (negative and positive) were found to be 20% in relation to arterial disease. It should be stressed that occlusions of the internal pudendal artery are not necessarily followed by a substantial decrease in the PBPI.

Conclusion

Blood pressure measurements may be helpful in diagnosing arterial insufficiency, but as a single diagnostic procedure, the ability of the test to exclude arterial insufficiency as a cause of erectile dysfunction is not satisfactory. It should further be stressed that penile blood pressure measurement does not tell anything about the condition of flow and, finally, that the measurement is done in the flaccid state. Detection of single arteries with the Doppler technique and evaluation of the appearance of the pulse curve seem promising in the diagnosis of arterial insufficiency.

Nocturnal Penile Tumescence

Periodic penile tumescence during sleep was originally described by Ohlmeyer and Brilmayer (1947). In healthy young adults, an ultradian rhythm of 90–120 min between episodes, which may last from 20 to 50 min, was found. Similar rhythm in the awake state may exist, but it is more-or-less suppressed by environmental conditions and may be interfered with by sexual activity or arousal. Other vegetative functions like frequency of respiration, heartbeat, and involuntary muscle contractions also exhibit phasic changes. During the dream phases of sleep, a pattern of rapid eye movements occurs (REM phase of sleep). In these periods, penile tumescence takes place (Fisher *et al.*, 1965; Jovanović, 1967a). No systematic studies of animal nocturnal erection exist, but scattered observations have led to the belief that the phenomenon also exists in the animal kingdom. In 1940, Halverson reported penile erection in male infants between the age of 3 and 20 months occurring in the awake state and during sleep at a relatively high frequency. This finding is in good concordance with the later-described dominance of REM-phase sleep in newborns. During intrauterine life, the male fetus may have penile erection, as is occasionally observed during amnioscopy.

The most extensive study has been done by Jovanović (1972), who in his monograph described 866 night studies of 211 normal subjects of a wide age range and 199 patients during 948 nights. Of the patients, 35 were suffering from sleep disturbances such as enuresis, sleepwalking, sleep talking, or pavor nocturnus, and 164 were suffering from "impotence." Unfortunately, the author did not define the latter term. Of the "impotent" patients, 55% were classified as psychiatric

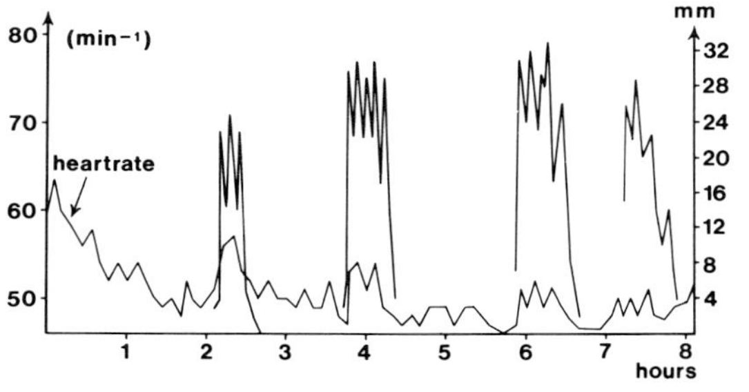

Figure 35. Nocturnal penile tumescence (NPT) and heart rate during eight hours' sleep in a healthy 30-year-old man with initial low heart rate. Four episodes of NPT are recorded. Right ordinate: increase in penile circumference. Cf. Figure 36. (Jovanović, 1972.)

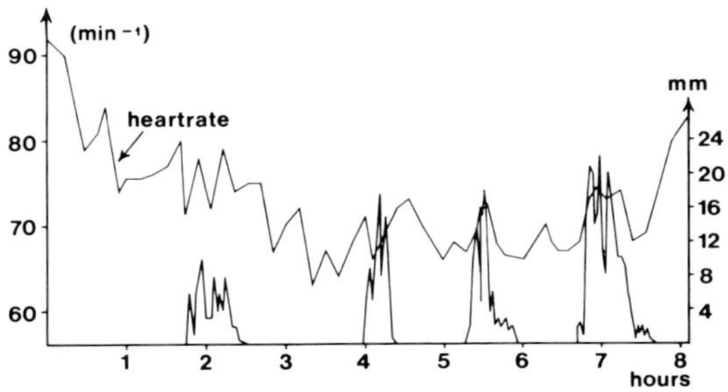

Figure 36. Nocturnal penile tumescence (NPT) and heart rate during eight hours' sleep in a healthy 25-year-old man with an initial heart rate of 94/min. The four erectile episodes are less "strong" than those seen in Figure 35. Right ordinate: increase in penile circumference. (Jovanović, 1972.)

patients with sleep disturbances, neuroses, depression, or schizophrenia. It was found that some disorder of sleep and disorders of sexual life coincided in most of the dysfunctional cases. Simultaneous recordings were made in the sleep laboratory of the electroenchepalogram (EEG), the electrooculogram (EOG), the electromyogram (EMG), the electrocardiogram (ECG), and the respirogram (resp).

Nocturnal penile tumescence (NPT) was recorded by applying a circular graphite transducer around the middle of the shaft of the penis. As can be seen in Table X, different types of transducers can be used to obtain a volumetric impression of tumescence. It is generally recommended that two circular transducers be used, as local disorders of the cavernous bodies may be encountered in defects in erection. Localized fibrosis or a Peyronie's body may prevent tumescence of a part of the erectile tissue and not necessarily the rest. Jovanović (1972) has described the first erection phase as lasting about 12 min, the second 19 min, the third 28 min, the fourth 27 min, the fifth 45 min, and the sixth, often interrupted by morning waking, from 10 to 50 min. The sixth phase is found only in individuals who sleep more than eight hours. The intervals between the REM–erection phases decrease during the night from 99 to 55 min. This pattern gives a total of more than 1½ hours of penile tumescence during sleep per night. The largest increase in penile volume is usually found in the period with the slowest heart rate (around 5 A.M.).

NPT is subject to influence negatively or positively by the quality of sleep, the somatic constitution, deprivation of sleep, anxiety, dream content, and dream symbolism. Good sleepers and good dreamers have the best erections as judged from the quantity of erections and the increase in circumference. Compared with asthenic and adipose men, men with athletic and pyknic body types show better erections. Also, the erection pattern is dependent on the "autonomic constitution." Figures 35 and 36 demonstrate the different heart rates of two subjects at the beginning of the recording and during sleep.

Table X. Comparison of Human Penile Measurement Techniques[a]

Type of transducer	Electrical specifications	Degree of sensitivity	Technical considerations	Reliability	Clinical considerations	Ease of use
I. Circumference methods						
A. Electromechanical strain gauges						
1. Binary strain gauge (Ohlmeyer *et al.*, 1947)	DC-low-voltage relay switch	Limited to binary output	Crude measurement device produced limited data.	Undetermined but probably reliable.	Portability and simplicity are positive clinical features.	Good
2. Barlow gauge (Barlow *et al.*, 1970; Modification: Laws, 1977)	DC-6-volt	Moderate	Rugged, light, and durable. Placement critical—problem of gauge ring slipping. Easy calibration.	Barlow gauge (very good) correlates with self-report. High reliability between and within sessions.	Unobtrusive. Convenient. Commercially available.	Excellent
3. Farrall erection sensor	No current in transducer	Low	Subject must be in upright position (because of gravity counterbalance)	Unreliable, susceptible to artifact (Laws, 1977).	Cumbersome.	Poor
B. Resistance strain gauges						
1. Mercury strain gauges (Fisher *et al.*, 1965; Bancroft *et al.*, 1966; Karacan, 1969; Rosen, 1973)	DC-low-voltage Can use AC display	Moderate	Durability range, 1–6 months.	Correlates reasonably well with self-report. Good test–retest reliability.	Very robust clinical tool. Can be worn under clothes. Least obtrusive.	Excellent

					Movement artifacts easily detectable. Can be positioned by subject.	
2. Graphite strain gauge (Jovanović, 1967b)	AC–DC 9 volts	Moderate	Thicker and more obtrusive than mercury. Less flexible. Separation problems during expansion.	Uncertain; no data available.	Obtrusiveness because of tensile strain. Similar to but less useful than mercury-in-rubber gauge.	Fair
II. Volumetric methods						
A. Water-filled penile plethysmograph (Fisher *et al.*, 1965)	No current in transducer	Low	Obtrusive because of weight.	No data available.	Size and bulk major drawbacks.	Poor
B. Air-filled penile plethysmographs (Freund *et al.*, 1965; McConaghy, 1967; Wagner & Brindley, 1980	No current: readout on pressure transducer	Very sensitive	Major problem with cuff attachment (Freund *et al.*, 1974). Movement artifacts. Temperature-sensitive.	High reliability within session. Poor between-session reliability. Valuable in research.	Most expensive and most obtrusive clinical method because of weight of transducer. Could elicit anxiety.	Poor

[a]Modified after Rosen and Keefe (1978).

Fatigue and earlier deprivation of sleep have a negative effect on NPT. The same applies to anxiety-producing situations. Figure 37 is an example of the first and second nights in a sleep laboratory, showing the negative effect of the unusual situation as experienced on the first night. This effect has led most researchers and clinical sleep laboratories to require three nights in the laboratory for recordings. As the recordings from the first two nights may serve as indicators of the period with the "best" erection, it is possible to look for this particular period during the third night and to make visual observation (or to photograph) the erection. Additionally, a judgment is made of the rigidity of the organ either by palpation or by measuring the resistance to buckling of the shaft. It is stated that previous sexual intercourse does not influence the erectile pattern as much as moderate doses of alcohol or medicine. It is generally recommended that the examination be done during nights following days during which no alcohol or drugs have been consumed.

The pattern of NPT from adolescence to about age 50 does not change significantly. In men older than 50, a reduction of the duration of erectile periods and the strength of erection is observed. The strength, however, may become reduced from age 40. This parameter decreases more dramatically in men over 60, the duration shortens, and the patterns become more like those of prepubertal boys. In men over 70, the periodicity is still maintained, but a reduction of strength and duration is marked in comparison with younger age groups.

Major interest has been given to NPT in the search for a tool that will differentiate between psychogenic and organic erectile failure. A man with a normal NPT who complains of impotence is supposed to suffer from "psychogenic impotence," while an abnormal NPT (reduced time of full tumescence and total time of NPT) is indicative of an organically based dysfunction. This discrimination was formulated on the examination, without any sophisticated diagnostic procedures, of nine patients (Fisher *et al.,* 1975), of whom three were diagnosed as psychic. Karacan *et al.* (1977) used a comparison of NPT from normal subjects and dysfunctional men, some of whom were nondiabetic and some of whom were diabetic. These researchers claimed that impotence with abnormal NPT and diabetes was organic and that impotence with normal NPT and the absence of

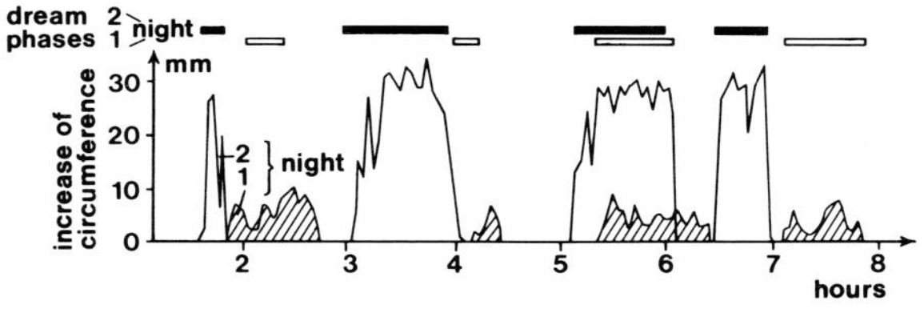

Figure 37. Comparison of NPT and dream phases (REM) from a healthy 22-year-old man during the first and second nights in a sleep laboratory. Duration and magnitude of tumescence increased from the first to the second night. (Jovanović, 1972.)

organic causes (although no sophisticated diagnostic procedures were applied) were to be considered psychogenic. The interpretation of these results is difficult, because neither the etiology nor the pathology of erectile failure in diabetic men is clear, because the etiology of psychogenic impotence is not fully known, and because "the existence of identifiable psychopathology not necessarily indicates the existence of a psychological cause of impotence" (Karacan, 1977).

In a later report, Karacan *et al.* (1978) compared the NPT and the penile blood pressure in 36 dysfunctional men selected for age in three groups: one with normal NPT, one with abnormal NPT, and one with diabetes and abnormal NPT. Unlike other investigators, they made use of the penile blood pressure *per se* and not the penile blood pressure index. Recalculating their figures into an index does not give any indication of gross arterial insufficiency such as is seen in atherosclerotic dysfunctional men.

More serious objections to the NPT as a solid differential diagnostic tool in erectile dysfunction is the possible miss of patients with the "steal syndrome" (p. 68), who may have completely normal and firm erections, and in young patients with arterial dysplasia, who may need a long time to achieve full erection.

Another serious problem in an uncritical application of NPT is the nonlinearity of tumescence and rigidity. The intracavernous pressure necessary to maintain the rigidity of the penis to such an extent that vaginal penetration is possible does not build up until after the full volume increase has occurred and the tunica albuginea (and possibly the cavernous tissue) is stretched. Figure 38 shows an experiment demonstrating the pitfall of volumetric (by measuring circumference) assessment of erection.

The newly proposed idea of a portable system for home use to assess NPT (Gonick and Kenepp, 1979) may be a method that gives false positive answers. Those patients who are able to achieve full tumescence, but not full rigidity, may be misdiagnosed as psychogenic. In this category are many patients with abnormal drainage conditions.

Conclusion

NPT is one of many tests that may add to a proper diagnosis of erectile dysfunction. It is imperative to conduct two or three nights' studies and to observe (or measure) the maximum tumescence for rigidity of the shaft. As a sole examination of differentiation between psychogenic and organic dysfunction, NPT is not valid.

Penile Blood Flow

In 1978, the Tokyo group and the Copenhagen group reported on the successful application of the xenon-washout technique as a measurement of blood

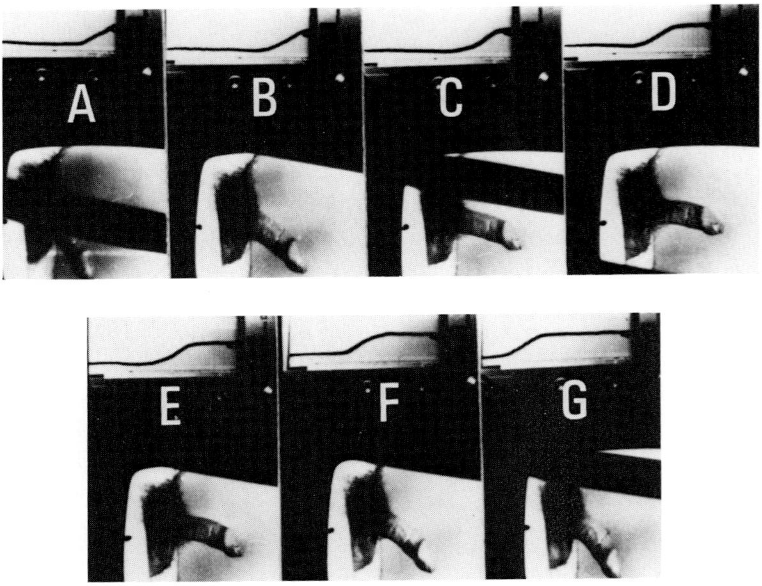

Figure 38. Illustration of an experiment carried out in a 24-year-old normal man. A to G are serial photos taken during the experiment of a pen-recording (top) and a videomonitor (bottom) connected to a TV camera placed to the right side of the standing man. A circular mercury strain gauge was placed around the shaft of the penis, and the upward deflection of the pen indicates an increase in the penile circumference. A to D are photos taken while the man was visually stimulated by an erotic filmstrip. It can be noted that at C, the maximum circumference had already been achieved, although full erection had not been accomplished, as judged from the penis-to-body angle. At D, the filmstrip was stopped, and although the erection (i.e., the rigidity or the intracavernous pressure) was subsiding (E to G), the circumference of the penis was unchanged. The experiment demonstrates that rigidity and circumference are not parallel and that detumescence (and decrease of circumference) occurs after the decrease of erection (i.e., intracavernous pressure). Thus, rigidity (and therefore the functional sexual capacity of the penis) cannot be evaluated via measurement of changes of circumference of the penis.

flow in the cavernous bodies in the flaccid state and during erection. Although applying almost identical procedures and obtaining values of blood flow of the same magnitude in flaccidity, their results during tumescence differed considerably. Shirai *et al.* (1978) found a dramatic increase in flow, while Wagner and Uhrenholdt (1978) reported a decreasing or unchanged flow.

When a deposit of radioactive xenon dissolved in sterile saline is placed in a tissue, it disappears, depending on the local blood flow as the rate-limiting factor. In a semilogarithmic plotting of the detected counts per minute, a linear (monoexponential) disappearance curve indicates a monocompartmental washout (Kety,

1949) and allows for a simple calculation of blood flow indicated as milliliters (blood) per minute per 100 g tissue ($ml \cdot min^{-1} \cdot 100g^{-1}$) (Lassen *et al.*, 1964):

$$PBF_{cc} = \frac{\ln 2 \cdot \lambda}{T_{1/2}}$$

where PBF_{cc} is the penile blood flow of the cavernous body, λ the blood-to-tissue partition coefficient, and $T_{1/2}$ the time taken to reach half the count of radioactivity left in the deposit. The method has proved to be of value in determination of the blood flow of several tissues and organs and is widely used for clinical and scientific purposes.

In this method 2–400 μCi Xe^{133} dissolved in sterile saline is injected without anesthesia into the lateral part of one of the cavernous bodies. When using a 27-gauge needle, only slight pain deriving from penetration of the skin is felt. No pain is experienced during the injection of the small volume into the erectile tissue. The needle is withdrawn after a short while, and slight finger pressure is applied to the site of injection to prevent bleeding with outflow of the radioactive solution. The patient is then fitted with a circular strain gauge and seated comfortably. The NaI-scintillation detector is placed 20–40 cm above the penis and directed so as to detect the maximum count of radioactivity from the deposit.

In the resting (flaccid) state a monoexponential curve is obtained, indicating a monocompartmental washout of radioactivity. In normal young men, values can be calculated ranging from 2.5 to 8 ml/min/100 g tissue in the flaccid state. To evaluate blood flow during erection, visual sexual stimulation is applied. The patient has to be carefully instructed as to the purpose and the course of the examination before the procedure is undertaken. Ideally, he should be effectively sheltered from the examiner and should also be fitted with ear protectors, as sounds easily disturb his ability to concentrate on the film material presented.

Figure 39A demonstrates the washout curve and circumference change in a 25-year-old normal man. The pattern is characterized by a monoexponential fall at rest and a change of slope when the visual stimulation is started. This pattern indicates that a slight decrease in outflow, sometimes temporarily down to zero, takes place during normal erection (see Chapter 3). When the stimulation stops, the disappearance rate increases at the time of penile detumescence, which is seen to have a first fast phase followed by a second slower one, often of considerable duration.

If a man with erectile dysfunction due to leakage from the cavernous bodies is examined by the xenon method, the pattern shown in Figure 39B can be found. During sexual stimulation, the outflow from the cavernous bodies increases, as no regulatory system is preventing the increase in outflow from the increase in pressure because of the abnormal leakage.

The basal flow in the flaccid state is the same as in normals. When measuring

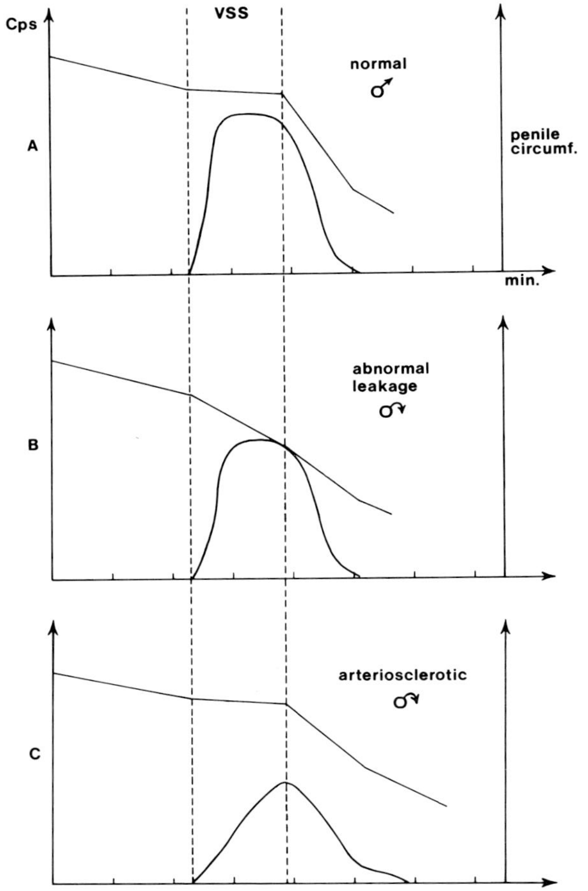

Figure 39. Simultaneous recording of penile circumference and radioactive Xenon[133] washout from the cavernous bodies before, during, and after visual sexual stimulation (VSS). Schematic representation (Cps = counts per sec). A. Depicts the normal condition with a modest washout of radioactivity in flaccidity, followed by a slight reduction in washout (outflow) with VSS during the tumescence and erection phases. At the end of stimulation, a sudden increase in washout occurs during detumescence. B. A washout curve from a dysfunctional man with abnormal leakage from the cavernous bodies. Characteristic increase in washout during sexual arousal leading to tumescence may sometimes be normal but not of sufficient rigidity because of leakage. C. The washout curve in a patient with arterial insufficiency may not differ from that of a normal person, except perhaps by a slower prestimulation washout. The increase in penile tumescence is prolonged and diminished.

the flow rate in patients with dysfunction due to arteriosclerosis, a low value in the flaccid state is found compared with that of normals (Figure 39C). During stimulation, a further reduction of flow occurs although the volume increase may be only modest. After stimulation, an increase is seen.

Arterial flow response to induced ischemia is a well-known phenomenon. A sluggish response may indicate arterial insufficiency. The postischemic test for the study of penile arterial response was introduced by Britt *et al.* (1971) and was revised by Kempczinski (1979). The configuration of the arterial pulse was obtained by the Doppler technique after 4 min of ischemia. The xenon-flow method has also been used for this purpose.

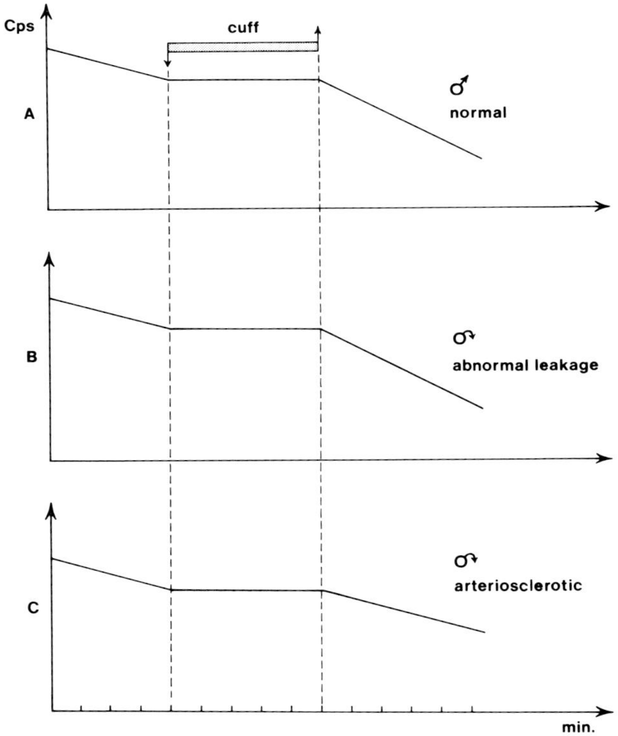

Figure 40. Schematic representation of postocclusive blood flow of the cavernous bodies measured by the xenon-washout method. Flow in flaccidity is measured 3–5 min before a cuff placed at the root of the penis is blown up to suprasystolic pressure and kept at this pressure for 5 min. During this period, no washout of the radioactivity occurs. After the release of the cuff pressure, the washout (flow), increases above the preocclusive value in A (normal) and B (venous leakage) as opposite to C, in which the flow is equal to or only slightly increased, indicating insufficient arterial response to ischemia. (Cps = counts per sec.)

A cuff placed around the root of the flaccid penis is filled with a pressure that is higher than the systemic systolic pressure and that is kept at this value for 5 min. The xenon curve flattens out, as no blood is drained off the erectile tissue during this period (Figure 40). When the pressure is released, the flow exceeds that of the basal state in flaccidity in normal men and in men who are dysfunctional for other reasons than arterial insufficiency. However, in dysfunctional arteriosclerotics, the postocclusive blood flow is similar to the basal flow found before the induced ischemia, indicating a decreased arterial response.

Two possible explanations can be given for the difference in the results by Shirai *et al.* and Wagner and Uhrenholdt. The Japanese researchers used a very short period of visual stimulation and measure in the period after stimulation. Also, they injected local anesthesia before the deposit of xenon. This may interfere with the neural regulation of the drainage system, preventing its closure.

Conclusion

The xenon-washout technique is a valuable diagnostic tool, as it may disclose abnormal leakages from the cavernous bodies during sexual stimulation. The postischemic test may be indicative of cases of arterial insufficiency.

Infusion Cavernosography

To obtain a picture of the cavernous spaces, their outline, and their drainage system, it is necessary to perform cavernosography. Traditionally, this is made by injection of a radio-contrast medium into one of the cavernous bodies followed by X-ray films.

In a normal subject, fine venous structures are seen around the compact and uniformly solid cavernous bodies. No contrast is seen in the glans. A cavernosogram performed in a case of priapism reveals no outlet from the cavernous body (Ebbehøj, 1975). If a large fistula is produced, as in the case of surgical treatment for priapism, normal cavernosography discloses its localization and size. If, however, smaller fistulas exist, they may not be revealed (Ebbehøj and Wagner, 1979). A slow infusion (2–5 ml/min) of a radio-contrast medium like Urografin® (sodium, meglumine diatrizoate) should be given by an infusion pump. Dilution of the contrast medium to half the commercial strength is necessary in order to prevent endothelial damage. The needle is inserted without anesthesia in the lateral side of one of the cavernous bodies. Its discomfort is equivalent to a venipuncture and the discomfort normally subsides in one or two minutes. Any pain experienced once the infusion is started may indicate wrong positioning of the tip of the needle. The infusion is started and the position of the needle is controlled on a monitor, preferably coupled to a videorecorder (Ebbehøj *et al.,* 1978).

Once the cavernous bodies are filled, the drainage system is seen (Figure

41A). As only the mobile part of the penis is shown, it is the drainage through the dorsal venous system that can be clearly defined. This system also drains the glans, and the possibility exists of some retrograde filling of the glans with contrast medium. Figures 42A and 42B demonstrate this possibility from two different postmortem experiments in which an ink-stained wax solution was infused into the cavernous bodies. It is not known whether the retrograde filling is a normal phenomenon or is due to a decreased function of the veins.

The patient rests on his side and the penis is slightly stretched with adhesive tape. A specially constructed needle with two canals gives the possibility of simultaneous recording of intracavernous pressure. Tumescence can be measured at the same time by use of a circular strain gauge placed immediately behind the corona glandis (Figure 41). Because of the incomplete system between the two cavernous bodies, both fill with contrast medium.

In order to obtain a picture of such abnormal drainage conditions as those described in Chapters 11 and 12 it is necessary to provoke an erection or the initiation of an erection. The patient is fitted with ear protectors, and a sexually stimulating filmstrip is shown on a TV monitor. This procedure usually produces a rapid response in younger men and may result in full erection with an increase of intracavernous pressure to nearly that of the mean arterial pressure. In patients older than 40, a slower and less pronounced response is common.

In men with supposedly normal erectile function who are being seen for other penile pathology, the contrast medium in draining veins disappears a few seconds after the initiation of the visual stimulation and often before any significant tumescence or increase in pressure occurs. No drainage or slight drainage is noted during the tumescence phase or during erection. When the stimulation ceases, the venous drainage system suddenly reappears before detumescence and the drop in pressure.

This method thus permits the study of the functional state of the draining system, which clearly seems to be regulated by the nervous system involved in the mechanism of erection.

In a recent study, the Copenhagen group has noted three different patterns that vary from the normal (Ebbehøj *et al.,* 1980):

1. The venous drainage decreases at the onset of stimulation, but tumescence and pressure increase are minimal. These cases suggest an arterial disorder with normal neural regulation.
2. The venous drainage is unaltered, and there is no change of volume and pressure, indicating that the stimulation has not been effective. The patient may have been unable to concentrate, partly because of the disturbing environment. Among these cases, some psychogenic patients are found.
3. The venous drainage system fades away at stimulation, with tumescence and pressure increasing only up to a certain point when the contrast

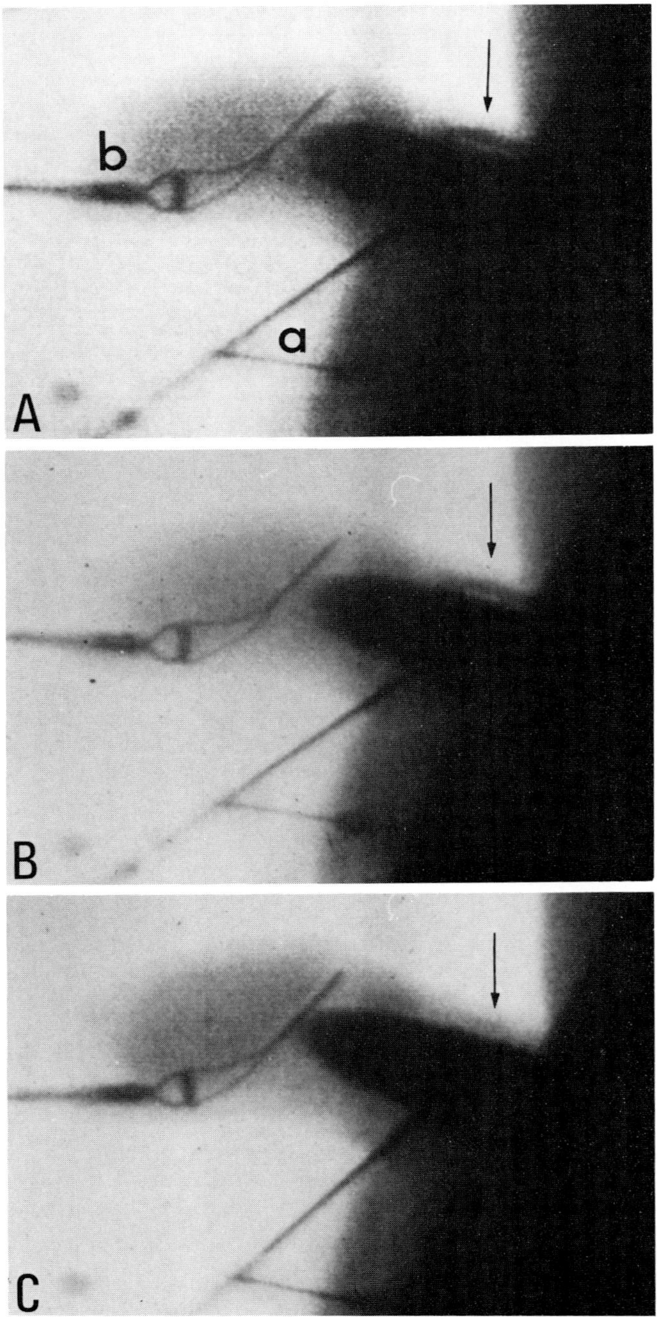
b
a
A
B
C

Figure 41. Photos of fluoroscopic examination videotaped during infusion cavernosography with simultaneous measurement of change of penile circumference and intracavernous pressure in a normal 29-year-old man. (a) indicates a needle with a double lumen, one infused with contrast medium, while the intracavernous space is connected to a pressure transducer through the other. (b) shows the mercury strain gauge applied proximally to the glans. A. During flaccidity. Arrow points to the contrast-filled venous draining system of the dorsum of the penis. B. Visual sexual stimulation (VSS) has begun, and a slight increase in the length of the cavernous bodies (in black) is noted. The arrow points to the modest thinning of contrast in the draining vein. C. Further tumescence has taken place during the continuing VSS, and the contrast medium of the draining system has disappeared (at arrow). The intracavernous pressure is 35 mm Hg. Regulation of the drainage system from the cavernous bodies is thus starting at an early stage of the tumescence phase of the erectile cycle.

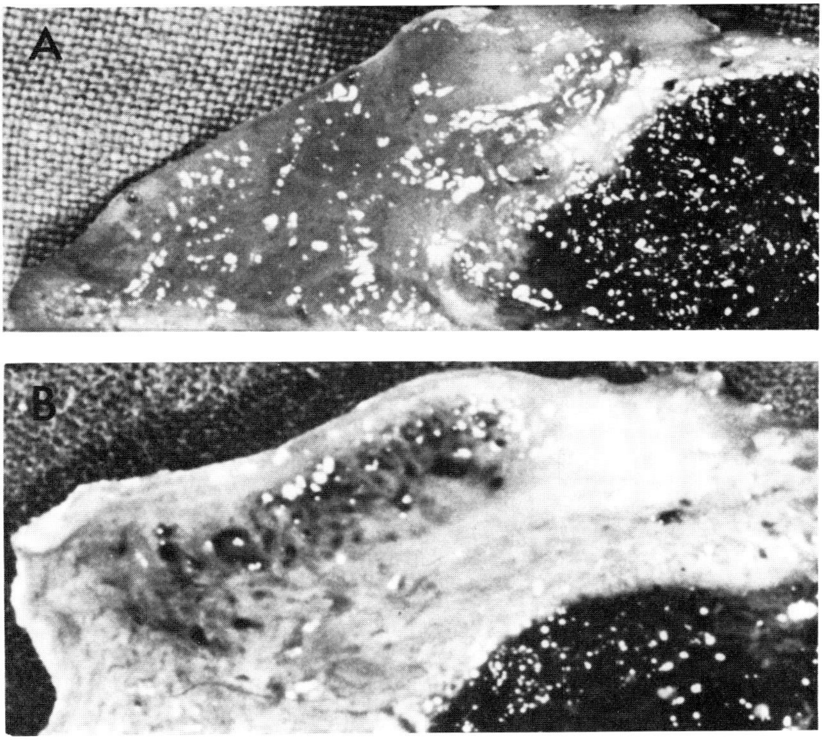

Figure 42. Photos of two postmortem specimens. The black area on the right side is the cavernous tissue; an ink-stained wax solution was injected into the cavernous bodies before dissection of the organ. To the left in both pictures is the spongiose tissue of the glans. No direct passage of fluid has occurred in the preparation. A. No stain is found in the glans. B. Some stain is seen in the glans. The passage has taken place through the communicating venous system distally on the dorsum of the penis but outside the tunica albuginea. The preparations prove that no direct communications exist between the cavernous and the spongiose bodies.

medium is seen leaving the cavernous bodies, sometimes in spurts synchronous with the pulse. These abnormal outlets may be seen at the border between the cavernous and spongiose corpora or at large communications to veins. In some patients, the leaking occurs at a low intracavernous pressure, while in others, the leakage is seen only at a higher pressure.

Conclusions

Cavernosography is a useful method in localization of defects of the cavernous bodies, but infusion cavernosography combined with visual sexual stimulation is necessary to detect abnormal function of the drainage system.

Thermography

Penile thermography as a diagnostic measure was suggested by Tordjman (1977) and was claimed to be of value in the diagnosis of arterial as well as venous causes for erectile dysfunction. The possibility of penile thermography as a detector of decreased arterial perfusion would render a rather simple screening procedure for such cases.

In a recent critical study, Lemaire *et al.* (1979) examined cases of erectile dysfunction and excluded all known organic etiologies except vascular. Twenty-nine men were then exposed to thermography, with four pictures taken in neutral temperature, and during and after cooling. In each patient, 16 sets of thermic data and 8 temperature gradients were studied. Arteriography was also carried out by use of the Seldinger technique (p. 123), and the results were classified as normal, or as medium or severe lesions of the arterial supply to the penis.

A study of 104 comparisons showed that none of the thermographic parameters allowed separation of patients with normal arteriograms from those with severe arterial damage. The authors concluded that penile thermography has no value in the selection of patients for arteriography.

Figure 43. Selective internal iliac arteriography, in a normal 31-year-old man depicting the left side of the arterial supply to the penis. A. Photo taken when contrast medium has reached the area where the single arteries to the penis branch off. (d) marks the distal segment of the internal pudendal artery (also called the *penile artery*) around the passage of the urogenital diaphragm (cf. Figure 49, upper arrow). (c) indicates the proximal part of the bulbar artery before it enters the spongiose body, while (b) points to the left deep penile artery where it pierces the crus of the left cavernous body. Also the beginning of the dorsal artery is seen at this point—cf. (b) in Figure 43B. B. Photo taken some seconds after A. The contrast medium has now filled the left dorsal artery (a) all the way to the glans. (b) points to where the deep artery pierces the tunica albuginea, and it can be seen that contrast material has filled a large part of the cavernous body (the cloudy area below the dorsal artery). Also, the bulbar part of the spongiose body is visible now as a solid, wide structure supplied by the bulbar artery (c).

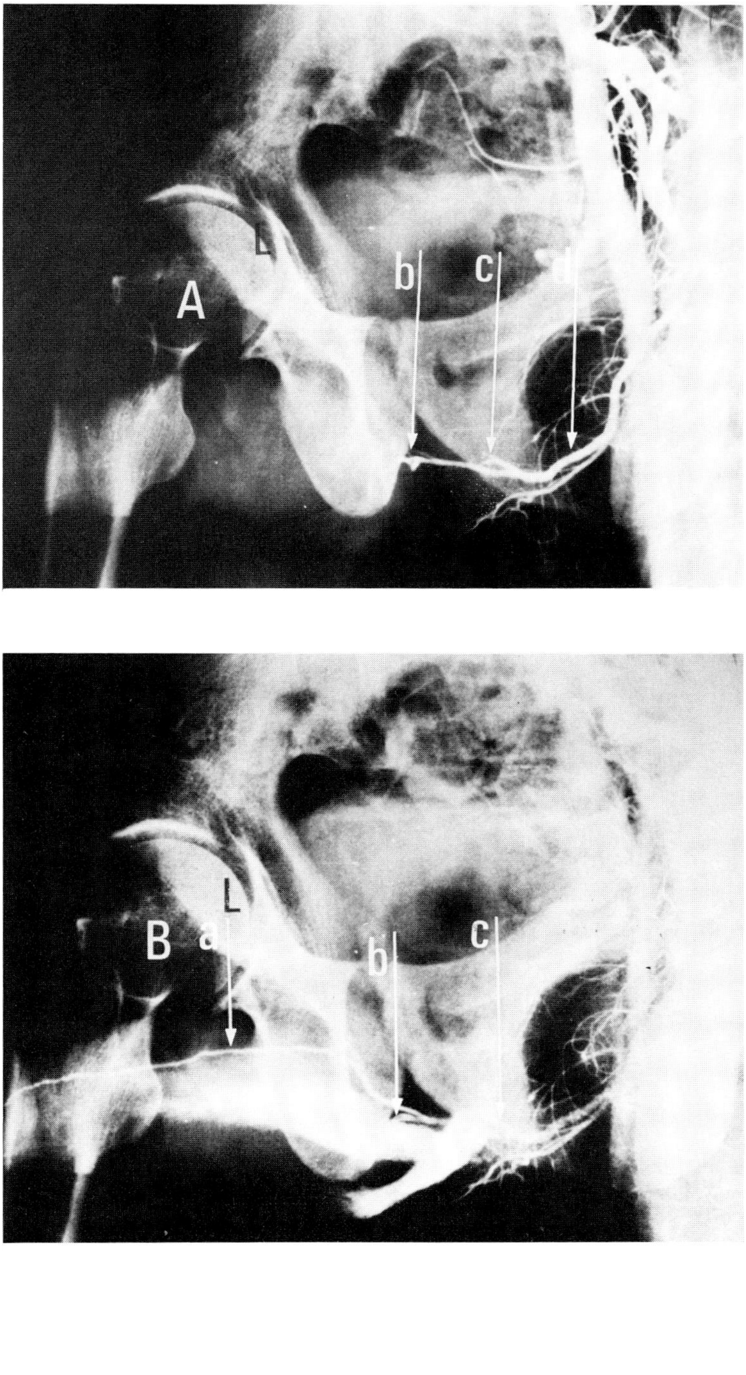
L
A
b
c
L
B
a
b
c

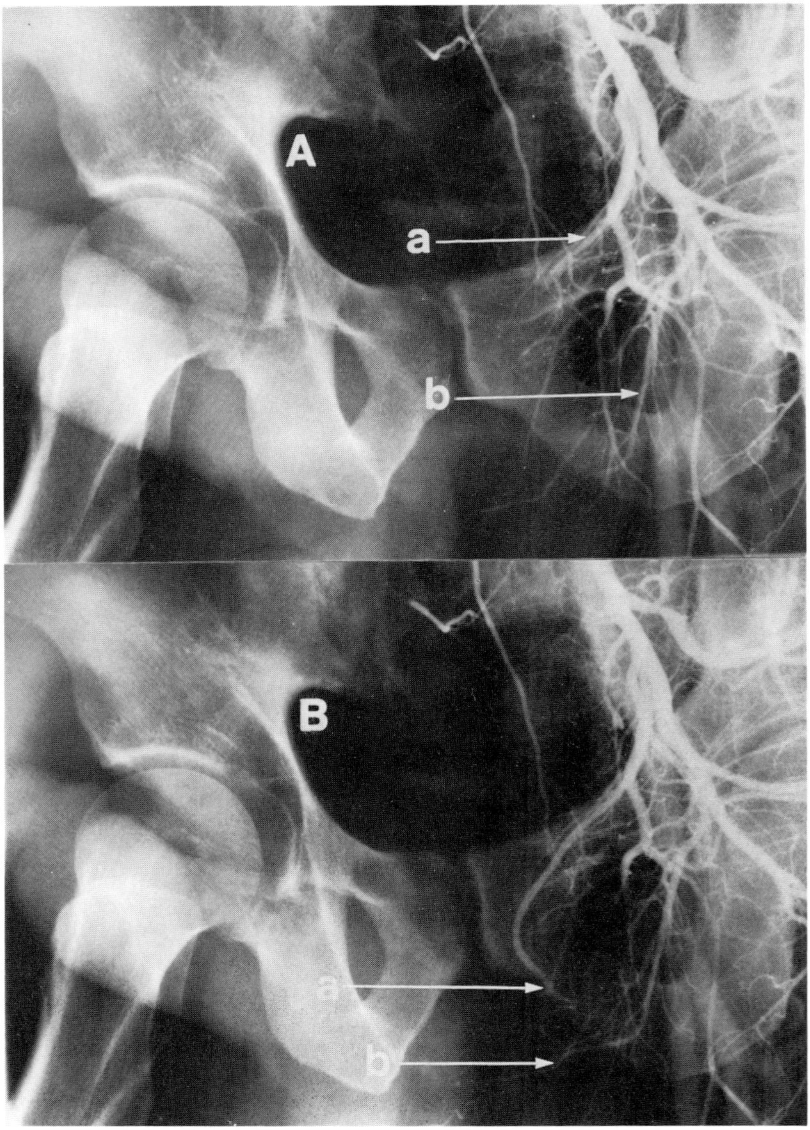

Figure 44. Left-side selective internal iliac arteriography in a 24-year-old man with primary erectile dysfunction. The right side displayed almost the same lack of normal arterial supply. The shadow of the penis is seen over the head of the right femur. A. Early filling of (a) the accessory pudendal artery and (b) the internal pudendal artery of the left side. B. Photo 2 sec after A. Further filling of accessory pudendal artery (a). Internal pudendal artery gives off perineal branches (b). C. Photo 2

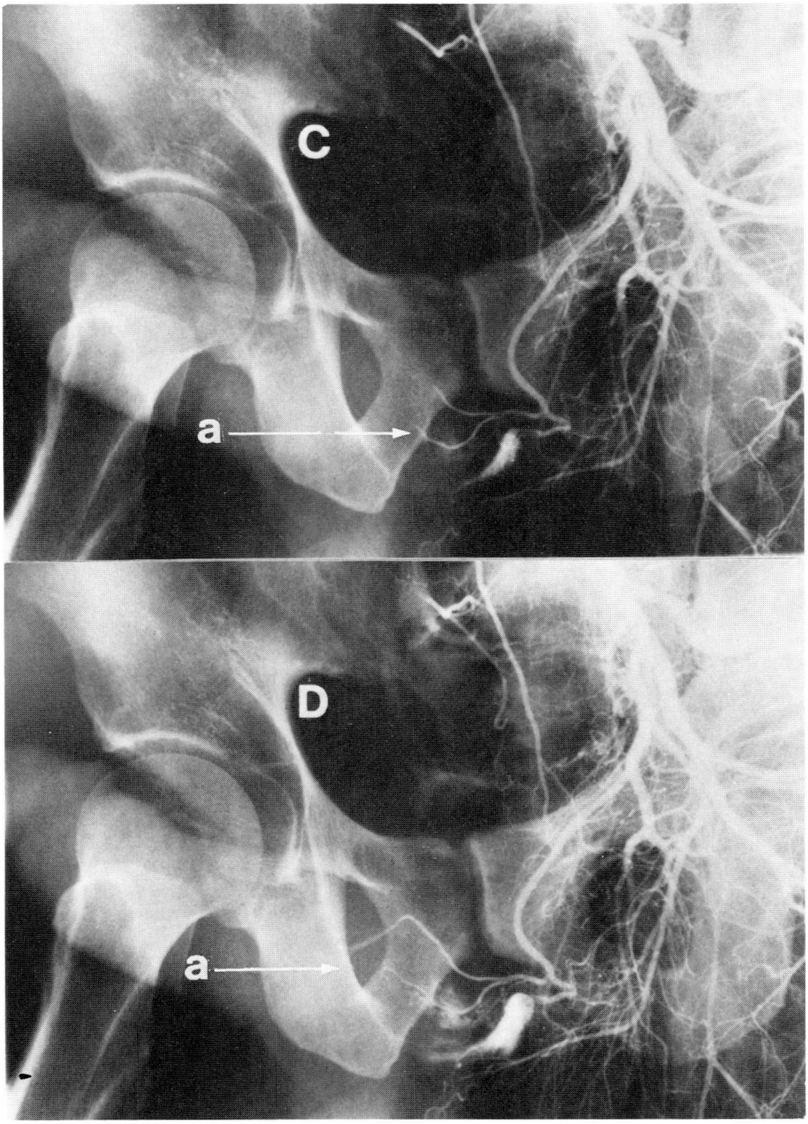

sec after B. Early filling of the three penile branches from the accessory pudendal artery (a). Bulbar shadow is clearly visible. D. Photo 2 sec after C. Further filling of dorsal, deep, and bulbar penile arteries (a). Although well calibrated, the filling from the accessory pudendal artery is delayed compared with that of the rest of the branches of the iliac artery.

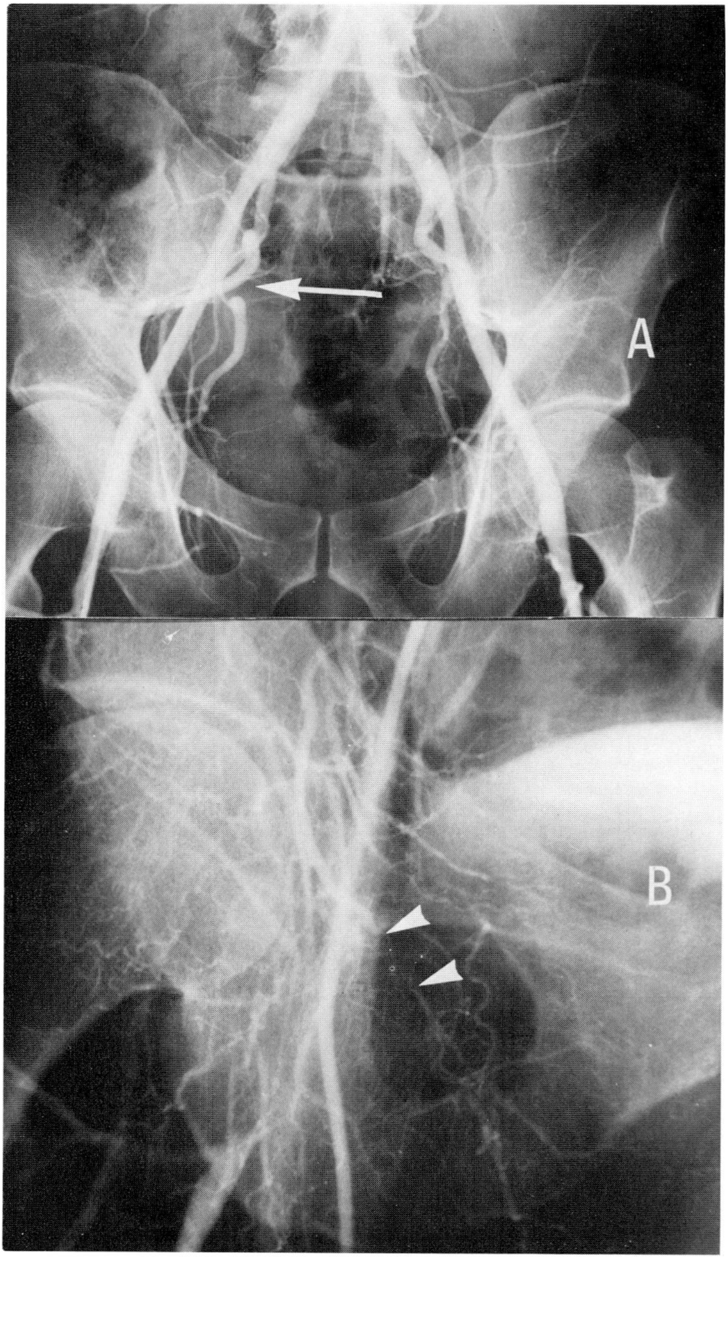
A
B

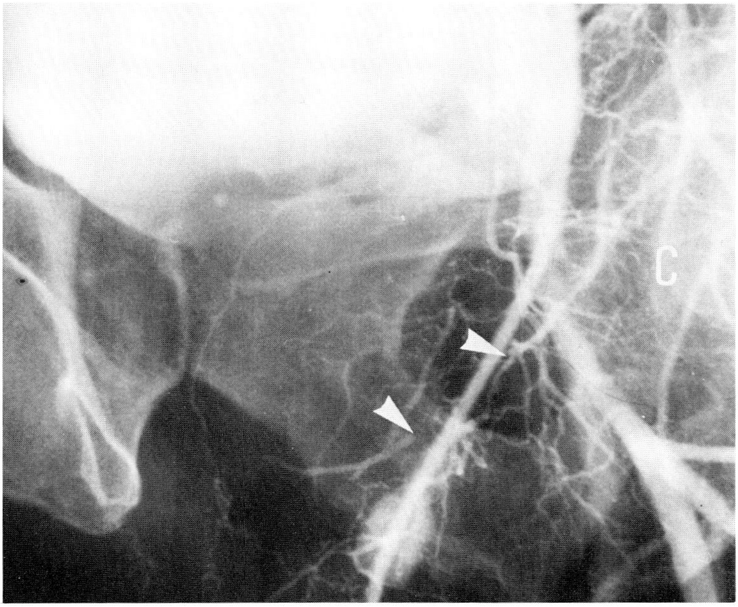

Figure 45. Arteriography in a 47-year-old man with a history of six years' insidious occurrence of erectile dysfunction. A. Total view of aortic bifurcation and iliac regions (a): occlusion of proximal part of right internal pudendal artery. B. Right selective internal iliac arteriography. Between the arrows can be seen the occlusion of the internal pudendal artery. C. Left selective internal iliac arteriography. The internal pudendal artery is occluded between the arrows.

Arteriography

Radiographic visualization and localization of atherosclerosis and thrombi around the aortic bifurcation and in the large vessels are a common finding. Branches from the internal iliac artery leading to the penis are not normally clearly defined, and the three penile branches (cf. Figure 5, Chapter 1) are not demonstrated.

Selective bilateral internal iliac arteriography (Ginestié *et al.*, 1976) or selective pudendal arteriography (Struyven *et al.*, 1979), sometimes combined with artificial erection (Michal and Pospichal, 1978), has revealed penile arteries. Full anesthesia is used, and the Seldinger technique for arterial perforation is applied. Insertion can be made via the left axillary artery or, better, through both the left and the right femoral arteries. The tip of the catheter is placed under fluoroscopic control, and an infusion of 30–40 ml contrast medium is given in 10 sec by use of a constant infusion pump. X-ray pictures are taken every second; usually, 20 pic-

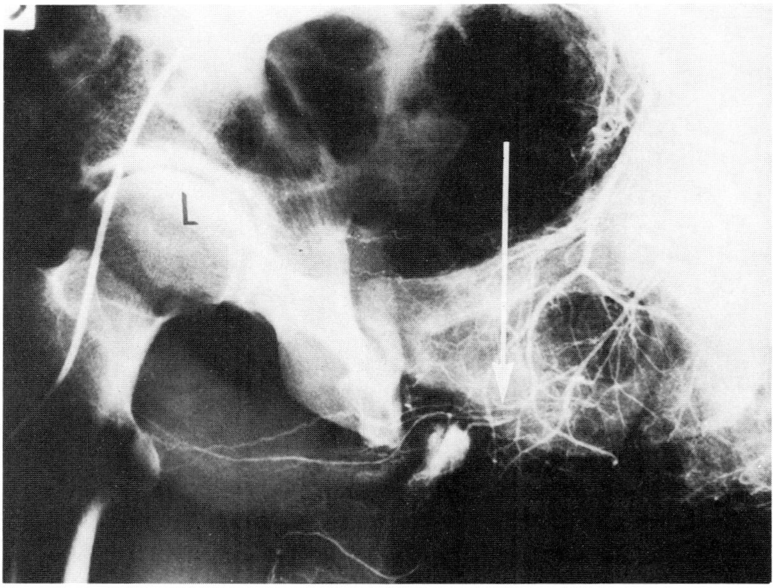

Figure 46. A 48-year-old man with a history of four months' complete lack of erection. Arteriography of the left side. The arrow points to an occlusion of the distal part of the internal pudendal artery. Collateral vessels have developed, and some arterial supply is seen in the penis, although it is insufficient for normal erectile function. The white area below and to the left of the arrowhead indicates the bulbus, which is sluggishly filling. (Figure courtesy of Dr. J. F. Huguet and Dr. C. Juhan, Marseilles, France.)

tures are exposed. The pictures are taken in oblique projection with the penis placed horizontally.

The introduction of "phalloarteriography" seems to have rendered a better picture of the penile arteries (Michal and Pospichal, 1978). The artificial erection is created by an infusion through a catheter into the cavernous tissue. This infusion stretches out the arterial system, providing a better possibility of studying local arterial lesions. During erection, the dorsal penile artery can be felt pulsating bilaterally. Michal and Pospichal (1978) found agreement between lack of pulsation and radiologically derived abnormal findings.

To produce the artificial (passive) erection, 45–160 ml of heparinized saline is infused per minute; 60% of this value is necessary to maintain erection. Recently, Virag (1980b) has pointed out that abnormal leakage from the cavernous bodies can be diagnosed by passive erection. The persistent high flow-rate that is necessary to maintain erection was found to be a good indicator of the occurrence of abnormal drainage responsible for erectile failure. An initial injection of acetylcholine or an alpha-blocker in saline into the arterial system prior to the contrast medium is used by some radiologists to enhance the possibility of localizing defects through vasodilation.

The finding that an increased flow is necessary to maintain erection has been taken by some as an indication of a high blood flow during normal erection. This highly artificial situation combined with general anesthesia cannot, however, be used as an argument against the low blood flow found by the xenon-washout technique during erection elicited by sexual stimulation with no use of anesthetics. Figures 44–49 show cases of arterial lesion localized by arteriography. The examination should be done only on strict indication. It should not be considered a routine test for erectile failure and should be used only where a convincing probability of arterial insufficiency exists.

Single-artery velocimetry (Doppler technique), as a screening technique for the necessity of performing arteriography, has been used by Juhan *et al.* (1978a). Further, they abolish the X-ray examination if the erectile dysfunction is selective

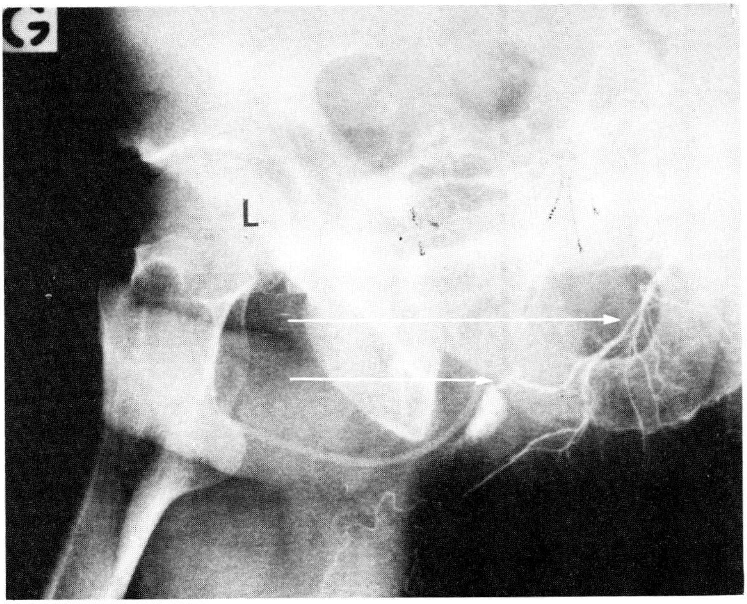

Figure 47. A 51-year-old man with one year's duration of difficulty in obtaining and maintaining erection. Left arteriography shows the mid-portion of the internal pudendal artery with stenosis (upper arrow) and filling of only the bulbar artery and the bulbus (lower arrow). (Figure courtesy of Dr. J. F. Huguet and Dr. C. Juhan, Marseilles, France.)

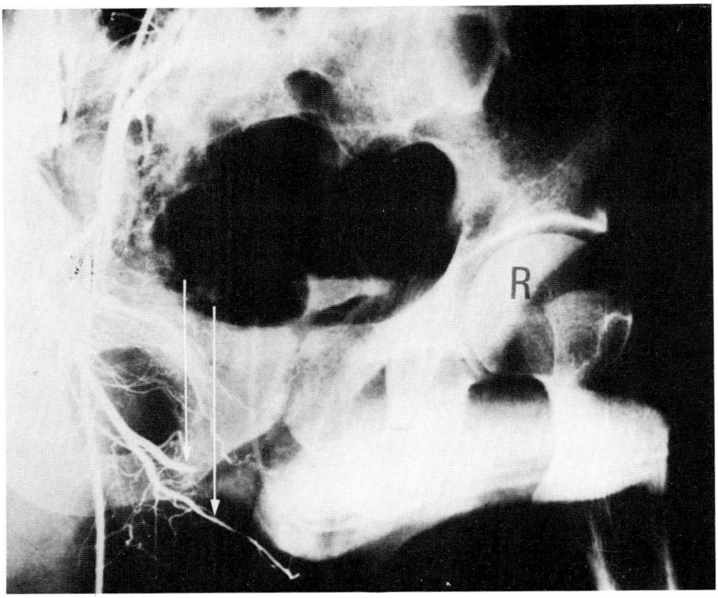

Figure 48. A 38-year-old man with 1½ year's history of inability to obtain penile rigidity. Tumescence was normal, although slow. Right-side arteriography shows very slow filling of the penile arteries on this side. The photo from the series shown here indicates a stenosis (at left arrow in the distal part) of the internal pudendal artery at the level of the urogenital diaphragm. The right arrow points to perineal arteries already filled at this time. Left-side arteriography was found to be normal. (Figure courtesy of Dr. J. F. Huguet and Dr. C. Juhan, Marseilles, France.)

with specific sexual partners, in cases of diabetes with demonstrated neuropathy, in patients with severe psychopathology, in patients with heart conditions, and where contraindications to general anesthesia exist. In a series of 100 consecutive cases of bilateral pudendal arteriography (mean age 44 years), 3% of the injections of contrast medium failed technically.

The Marseille group (Juhan *et al.,* 1978b) has analyzed arteriograms in 100 men. This analysis has led them to identify lesions with a characteristic topographic localization and has led them to suggest a "urogenital diaphragm syndrome." They divided the internal pudendal artery into three segments: (I) a proximal segment (up to the obturator foramen) where isolated lesions rarely are seen; (II) a mid-segment passing through Alcock's canal; and (III) a distal segment traversing the urogenital diaphragm (see Figure 5, Chapter 1).

In 15% of the 100 men studied, a localized lesion was found in Segment II, often bilaterally, while 25% of the arterial lesions were localized in Segment III and most often were unilateral. In 10%, lesions were found in both segments.

It seems logical to assume that a distally placed lesion may produce erectile dysfunction even when occurring unilaterally, while more proximal lesions more often have to be present on both sides to produce the erectile dysfunction (cf. findings demonstrated in Figure 24, Chapter 5).

In younger patients (below age 40) and nondiabetic men, a typical lesion will be found unilaterally in Segment II; hence the proposition of the new syndrome, as the authors suggested that extrinsic vascular compression may occur as the artery passes through the fibrous and muscular structures of the urogenital diaphragm.

In the 30 cases of Michal and Pospichal (1978), all patients showed various degrees of narrowing and obliteration of either the pudendal or the penile arteries or their peripheral branches. Sometimes, a stenotic area was bypassed by collateral vessels, often from the internal obturator or caudal vesical arteries. In four control studies (cases of psychogenic erectile failure), no pathology was found at arteriography. In their monograph, Ginestié and Romieu (1976) described the examination of 250 dysfunctional men and maintained that 25% showed pathology. They did not describe the composition or the selection of their patient group.

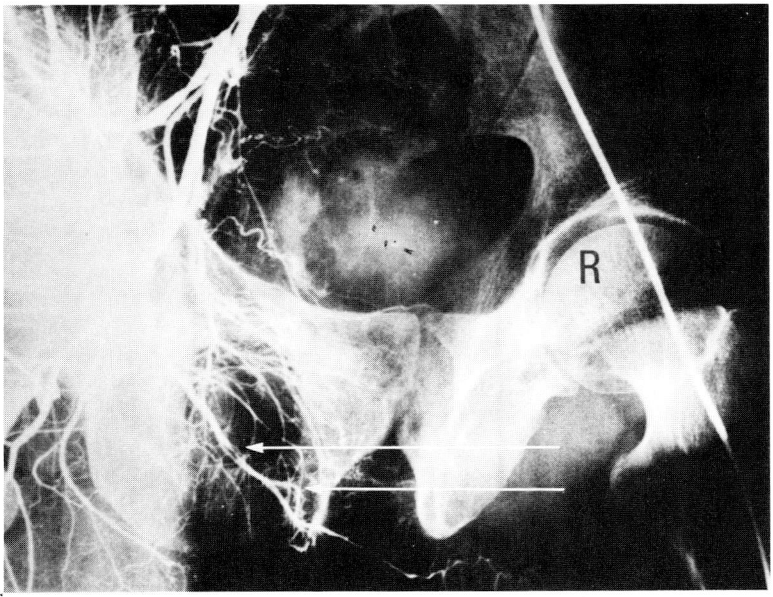

Figure 49. A 42-year-old man with a history of one year's erectile dysfunction making vaginal coitus impossible. The photo shows right-side arteriography with complete occlusion of the penile arteries (lower arrow) and severe distal stenosis of the internal pudendal artery. Left-side arteriography (not shown) gave a similar picture.

Conclusion

A series of new diagnostic procedures has developed during the last 10 years. Although it is preferable to make use of noninvasive techniques, it is rarely possible to avoid invasive radiological investigations if the underlying lesion is to be localized. If more simple noninvasive methods are used in the same patient, however, they will give a good indication of whether to continue with more invasive methods like cavernosography and/or arteriography.

References

Abelson, D. (1975). Diagnostic value of the penile pulse and blood pressure: A doppler study of impotence in diabetics. *The Journal of Urology, 113*, 636–639.

Bancroft, J. H. J. (1976). Evaluation of the effects of drugs on sexual behaviour. *British Journal of Clinical Pharmacology, Supplement,* 83–90.

Bancroft, J. H., Jones, H. G., and Pullan, B. P. (1966). A simple transducer for measuring penile erection with comments on its use in the treatment of sexual disorder. *Behavior Research and Therapy, 4*, 239–241.

Barlow, E. H., Becker, R., Leitenberg, H., and Agras, W. S. (1970). A mechanical strain gauge for recording penile circumference change. *Journal of Applied Behavior Analysis, 3*, 73–76.

Barry, J. M., and Hodges, C. V. (1978). Impotence: A diagnostic approach. *The Journal of Urology, 119*, 575–578.

Blaivas, J. G., O'Donnell, T. F., Gottlieb, P., and Labib, K. B. (1980). Comprehensive laboratory evaluation of impotent men. *The Journal of Urology, 124*, 201–204.

Britt, D. B., Kemmerer, W. T., and Robinson, J. R. (1970). Penile blood flow determination by mercury strain gauge plethysmography. *Investigative Urology, 8*, 673–678.

Canning, J. R., Lloyd, F. A., and Cottvell, T. L. C. (1963). Genital vascular insufficiency and impotence. *Surgical Forum, 14*, 298–299.

Ebbehøj, J. (1975). A new operation for priapism. *Scandinavian Journal of Reconstructive Surgery, 8*, 241–242.

Ebbehøj, J., and Wagner, G. (1979). Insufficient penile erection due to abnormal drainage of cavernous bodies. *Urology, 13*, 507–510.

Ebbehøj, J., Uhrenholdt, A., and Wagner, G. (1978). Infusion-cavernosography in the human in the unstimulated and stimulated situations and its diagnostic value. Presented at the *First International Conference on Vasculogenic Impotence,* New York.

Ebbehøj, J., Uhrenholdt, A., Metz, P., and Wagner, G. (1980). Preliminary results from the Copenhagen Impotence Study Group. Presented at the *Second International Conference on Vasculogenic Impotence,* Monaco, Oct. 10–12.

Edwards, A. E., and Husted, J. R. (1976). Penile sensitivity, age, and sexual behavior. *Journal of Clinical Psychology, 32*, 697–700.

Ellenberg, M. (1971). Impotence in diabetes. *Annals of Internal Medicine, 75*, 213–219.

Engel, G., Burnham, S. J., and Carter, M. F. (1978). Penile blood pressure in the evaluation of erectile impotence. *Fertility and Sterility, 30*, 687–690.

Fisher, C., Gross, J., and Zuch, J. (1965). Cycle of penile erection synchronous with dreaming (REM) sleep. *Archives of General Psychiatry, 12*, 27–45.

Fisher, C., Schiavi, R., Lear, H., Edwards, A., Davis, D. M., and Witken, A. P. (1975). The assessment of nocturnal REM erection in the differential diagnosis of sexual impotence. *Journal of Sex and Marital Therapy, 1*, 277–289.

Freund, K., Sedlacek, F., and Knob, K. (1965). A simple transducer for mechanical plethysmography of the male genital. *Journal of Experimental Analysis of Behavior, 8*, 169–170.

Freund, K., Langevin, R., and Barlow, D. (1974). Comparison of two penile measures of erotic arousal. *Behavior Research and Therapy, 12*, 355–359.

Gaylis, H. (1978). The assessment of impotence in aorto-iliac disease using penile blood pressure measurement. *Suid-Afrikaanse Tydskrift vir Chirurgie, 16*, 39–46.

Geer, J. H. (1976). Genital measure: Comments on their role in understanding human sexuality. *Journal of Sex and Marital Therapy, 2*, 165–174.

Ginestié, J., Ginestié, J.-F., and Romieu, A. (1976). Arteriographie des arteres honteuses internes revascularisation des corps caverneux dans les impuissances d'origine vasculaire. *Journal de Urologie et Nephrologie (Paris), 82*, 509–510.

Ginestié, J.-F, and Romieu, A. (1976). *L'Exploration radiologique de l'impuissance*. Paris: Maloine, S. A.

Gonick, P., and Kenepp, D. (1979). Home monitoring of penile tumescence for erectile dysfunction. Initial Experience. *Urology, 14*, 261–264.

Graber, B. (1979). Classification of erectile failure. Paper presented at the *IV World Congress of Sexology,* Mexico.

Jersild, M., and Lauritzen, E. (1957). Sensibilité vibratoire chez les diabètiques. *Le Diabète, 6*, 237–241.

Jovanović, U. J. (1967a). Erektionen im Schlaf. *Archiv für Neurologie und Psychiatrie, 210*, 220–237.

Jovanović, U. J. (1967b). A new method of phallography. *Confinia Neurologica, 29*, 299–312.

Jovanović, U. J. (1972). *Sexuelle Reaktionen und Schlafperiodik bei Menschen: Ergebnisse Experimenteller Untersuchungen*. Ferdinand Enke Verlag, Stuttgart.

Juhan, C. M., Jouven, C., and Fredenucci, P. (1978a). Doppler velocimetry of penile arteries and diagnosis of arteriogenic impotence. Presented at the *First International Conference on Vasculogenic Impotence,* New York.

Juhan, C. M., Huguet, J. F., Clerissi, J. A., and Courjavet, P. (1978b). Classification of lesions of the internal pudendal arteries. Presented at the *First International Conference on Vasculogenic Impotence,* New York.

Karacan, I. (1969). A simple and inexpensive transducer for quantitative measurements of penile erection during sleep. *Behavior Research Methods and Instrumentation, 1*, 251–252.

Karacan, I. (1970). Clinical value of nocturnal erection in the prognosis and diagnosis of impotence. *Medical Aspects of Human Sexuality, 4*, 25–34.

Karacan, I. (1977). Advances in the psychophysiological evaluation of male erectile impotence. *Weekly Psychiatry Update Series 43.*

Karacan, I., Scott, F. B., Salis, P. J., Attia, S. L., Ware, J. C., Altinel, A., and Williams, R. L. (1977). Nocturnal erections, differential diagnosis of impotence and diabetes. *Biological Psychiatry, 12*, 373–380.

Karacan, I., Ware, J. C., Dervent, B., Altinel, A., Thornby, J. I., Williams, R. L., Kaya, N., and Scott, F. B. (1978). Impotence and blood pressure in the flaccid penis: Relationship to nocturnal penile tumescence. *Sleep, 1*, 125–132.

Kempczinski, R. F. (1979). Role of the vascular diagnostic laboratory in the evaluation of male impotence. *The American Journal of Surgery, 138*, 278–282.

Kety, S. (1949). Measurement of regional circulation by the local clearance of radioactive sodium. *American Heart Journal, 38*, 321–326.

Kolářský, A., and Madlafousek, J. (1977). Variability of stimulus effect in the course of phallometric testing. *Archives of Sexual Behavior, 6*, 135–141.

Lassen, N. A., Lindbjerg, I. F., and Munck, O. (1964). Measurement of blood flow through skeletal muscle by intramuscular injection of Xenon-133. *Lancet, II*, 686–688.

Laws, D. R. (1977). A comparison of the measurement characteristics of two circumferential penile transducers. *Archives of Sexual Behavior, 6*, 45–51.

Lemaire, A., Besson, P., Dehaene, J. L., Buvat-Herbaut, M., and Buvat, J. (1979). Lack of correlations between penile thermography results and pelvic arteriography in 29 cases of erectile impotence. Presented at the *IV World Congress of Sexology,* Mexico.

Lundberg, P. O. (1978). Sexual function in men with neurological disorder. In E. S. E. Hafez (Ed.), *Human Semen and Fertility Regulation in Men.* St. Louis: C. V. Mosby.

McConaghy, N. (1967). Penile volume changes to moving pictures of male and female nudes in heterosexual and homosexual males. *Behavior Research and Therapy, 5*, 43–48.

Metz, P., and Bengtsson, J. (1981). Penile blood pressure. *Scandinavian Journal of Urology and Nephrology,* in press.

Michal, V., and Pospichal, J. (1978). Phalloarteriography in the diagnosis of erectile impotence. *World Journal of Surgery, 2*, 239–248.

Newman, H. F. (1970). Vibratory sensitivity of the penis. *Fertility and Sterility, 21*, 791–793.

Ohlmeyer, P., and Brilmayer, H. (1947). Periodische Vorgänge im Schlaf. *Pflügers Archiv für Gesammte Physiologie, 249*, 50–55.

Ohlmeyer, P., Brilmayer, H., and Hüllstrung, H. (1947). Periodische Vorgänge im Schlaf. *Pflügers Archiv für Gesammte Physiologie, 248*, 559–560.

Rosen, R. C. (1973). Suppression of penile tumescence by instrumental conditioning. *Psychosomatic Medicine, 35*, 509–513.

Rosen, R. C., and Keefe, F. J. (1978). The measurement of human penile tumescence, *Psychophysiology, 15*, 366–376.

Shirai, M., Ishii, N., Mitsukwa, S., Matsuda, S., and Nakamaru, M. (1978). Hemodynamic mechanism of erection in the human penis. *Archives of Andrology, 1,* 345–349.

Steiness, I. (1957). Vibratory perception in normal subjects. *Acta Medica Scandinavica, 158*, 315–327.

Struyven, J., Gregoir, W., Gionnakopoulos, X., and Wauters, E. (1979). Selective pudendal arteriography. *European Urology, 5*, 233–242.

Tordjman, G. (1977). Nouvelles acquisitions en pathologie vasculaire dans les dysfonctions erectiles de l'homme. *Cahiers de Sexologie Clinique, 3*, 19–27.

Vacek, J., and Lachman, M. (1977). Bulbokavernozni reflex u diabetiku s poruchou erektivitý: Klinicka a elektromyograficka studie. *Casopis lekaru ceskych, 116*, 1014–1015.

Velcek, D., Sniderman, K. W., Vaughan, E. D., Jr., Sos, T. A., and Muecke, E. C. (1980). Penile flow index utilizing a doppler pulse wave analysis to identify penile vascular insufficiency. *The Journal of Urology, 123*, 669–673.

Virag, R. (1980a). L'Exploration doppler de l'impuissance. *Angeiologie, 32*, 115–122.

Virag, R. (1980b). Presented at the *Second International Conference on Vasculogenic Impotence,* Monaco, Oct. 6–10.

Wagner, G. (1976). *Physiological Responses of the Sexually Stimulated Male in the Laboratory.* 16 mm color film. Copenhagen/New York.

Wagner, G. (1979). A differential diagnostic approach to erectile dysfunction. Presented at *IV World Congress of Sexology,* Mexico.

Wagner, G., and Brindley, G. S. (1980). The effect of atropine, alpha and beta blockers upon human penile erection: A controlled pilot study. In A. Zorgniotti and G. Rossi (Eds.), *Vasculogenic Impotence.* Springfield, Ill.: Charles C Thomas.

Wagner, G., and Uhrenholdt, A. (1978). Blood flow measurement by the clearance method in the human corpus cavernosum in the flaccid and erect states. Presented at the *First International Conference of Vasculogenic Impotence,* New York.

Weiss, A. D. (1971). Sensory functions. In J. E. Birren (Ed.), *Handbook of Aging and the Individual.* Chicago: University of Chicago Press.

CHAPTER 9

Psychotherapy of Erectile Failure

RICHARD GREEN

Introduction

The psychological treatments for erectile dysfunction are varied, probably because of their mixed record of success. But in fairness to those therapists who have attempted cures (and those patients who expected them), the mediocrity of results may be due to mixed etiologies: psychogenic and organic. On the other hand, clinicians are not typically hell-bent on systematic, crossover, experimental treatment designs. This wariness (or scorn, depending on the clinician) has not helped the psychotherapy "lobby" and makes scientific evaluation of treatment reports difficult.

To bring some semblance of order to this chapter, therapies are grossly categorized into an overriding approach, for example, individual versus group, psychodynamic versus behaviorist, and hypnotherapeutic versus mechanical. Some reports veer toward the anecdotal; some are experimental.

Psychoanalytically Oriented Individual Therapy

Here, the premise is that the erectile disorder represents an underlying unconscious conflict. The erectile dysfunction is seen as a neurotic defense against the emergence of conflicts noted in Chapter 6. Often, theory has it that parents who fear the child's sexual responses to them during the oedipal period, or those who are sexually competitive with their same-sex child, raise children who view subsequent sexual relationships as threatening (Bieber, 1974).

Three case reports by Layman (1972) illustrate the Freudian notion that erectile failure is the result of unconscious fears centering on the oedipus complex. Resolution of these fears through a gradual interpretive process was reported as successful. Erectile failure was seen as resulting from the spouse's being unconsciously perceived as an incestuous sex object, that is, as someone with whom one should be emotionally, but not sexually, close. Other psychodynamic orientations, rather than focusing on oedipal problems, look at general aspects of the interpersonal relationship (cf. Salzman, 1972; Kaplan, 1974; Gill and Temperlay, 1974; Hastings, 1971). Here, the dysfunction is seen as an expression of anger against the partner. Other clinicians underscore the importance of underlying depression (Proctor, 1973; Goldberg, 1973). The dysfunction is seen as only part of a constellation of problems centering on the individual's feelings of incompetence and lack of power. According to these clinicians, when the male examines the roots of these feelings and takes a more active role in life, both depression and erectile failure disappear.

An evaluation of psychoanalytic versus briefer therapy was attempted by O'Connor and Stern (1972). They looked, retrospectively, at results obtained during a 17-year clinical treatment period for 35 males with erectile problems. Psychoanalysis consisted of four sessions per week for a minimum of two years. This therapy had an overall improvement rate of 77% compared with only 46% for those receiving briefer therapy. However, Reynolds (1977) pointed out that the groups were not matched on a variety of characteristics and that the investigators noted that "patients who were analyzed evidenced less illness than those who received psychotherapy." This point is especially relevant in that the degree of concurrent psychopathology was found to be an important prognostic indicator.

Brief Couple and Individual Counseling

These approaches are oriented toward information giving, psychological support, and reassurance. An important concept, "performance anxiety," was advanced by Masters and Johnson (1970) (as noted in Chapter 6). Males become so concerned about the outcome of the sexual interaction that they fail to attend to erotic stimulation and other aspects of the sexual experience. This attitude must be reversed. Earlier, Tuthill (1955) designed therapy to help the male concern himself with experiencing and enhancing sexual pleasure and specifically advocated the use of erotic fantasies. Testosterone implants and various stimulants were also prescribed in some cases. Treatment evaluation was based on postal inquiries, and, although many men did not return the questionnaire, of the 148 respondents, 88% reported "satisfaction" with treatment.

A study that applied statistical analysis to prognostic indicators was that of Johnson (1965b), which included follow-up data for 62 men. Erectile dysfunction was the chief complaint of 40. The primary study aim was to describe and analyze the "natural course of male sexual disorders." The prognosis for all male sexual disorders, with or without treatment, was found to be poor, with two-thirds unchanged at six years' follow-up. Less that 17% were cured, and only 17% improved. Outcome results were better for men with erectile dysfunction compared with an ejaculatory disorder: nearly two-fifths of men with erectile disorder improved, compared with one-fourth of those with an ejaculatory disorder. Interestingly, 2 of 12 who received testosterone therapy and 11 of 21 who received "superficial" psychotherapy, counseling, or group therapy were also improved. Although the improvement rate for the treated cases was higher, the researcher acknowledged the possibility of pretreatment group differences. A history of successful coitus prior to the onset of the potency disorder was associated with a better prognosis, particularly for men with erectile dysfunction who developed the disorder during a recent engagement or marriage. However, late-onset dysfunction was a poor prognostic indicator, particularly when the disorder developed gradually during the marital experience.

In an interesting additional note, Johnson pointed out, "if disorders of sexual potency are largely psychogenic in nature, the improvement rate (even with treatment) does not even approach the spontaneous remission rate associated with neurotic states." Johnson suggested that "constitutional factors" in the etiology of these disorders are responsible for this poor improvement rate.

The erectile problems of 31 males were treated by Cooper (1968). Patients were divided into two groups: "acute onset impotence" and "insidious onset impotence." Treatment spanned at least 20 biweekly sessions over a period of about a year and consisted of an individually styled combination of progressive muscular relaxation, the provision of an "optimal" sexual environment, sex education, and psychotherapy. Joint interviews with the sexual partner were encouraged during the sex-education and "optimal" environment phases. Of the 31 men, 13 (42%) were rated as "cured" or "improved." Acute and insidious onset patients differed. Nearly 90% of the acute-onset males, compared with only 25% of the insidious-onset males, reported improvement.

Results of brief "urologic counseling" were reported by Finkel and Thompson (1972). Here, men were told that they had a "mild prostatitis," which the clinicians felt was less psychologically damaging news than when the men thought that their erectile disorder was purely psychogenic. They were told to increase their fluid intake, were given sulfonamide, and were reassured during subsequent visits that the prostatitis was improving. Then they were told they could resume intercourse on one occasion under relaxed conditions. Of the 84 men who completed therapy and follow-up, 60% had "sufficient improvement."

The pioneering and widely acclaimed example of couple sex therapy is that of Masters and Johnson (1970): 32 couples were treated in which the chief male complaint was "primary erectile dysfunction," plus 213 couples in which the male complaint was "secondary erectile dysfunction." Those men with primary erectile dysfunction had been unable to obtain or sustain an erection to the point of satisfactory coitus during both initial and subsequent "coital attempts." While many earlier-occurring factors were postulated as etiological (as noted in Chapter 6), the treatment format focused on the immediate causes within the couples' present sexual relationship. These included the man's "fear of performance" and the resultant "spectator role" that he assumed, plus his partner's concerns about her own sexual adequacy. The male's preoccupation with "willing an erection" was addressed. This results in increased anxiety and makes the male a *spectator* to his own sensual experience rather than a *participant* in it.

Treatment consisted of educational presentations, therapy discussions, and couple exercises. The couple met daily with a male and female sex therapy team over a two-week period in a setting away from their home environment. To reduce anxiety over performance, the couple were directed to refrain from coital attempts during the first days of treatment, during which they were instructed to engage in "sensate focus." This consists of exercises in which the partners reciprocally caress body areas other than the genitals or the female breasts. In this "nondemand situation," erection may occur. However, the couple are interdicted from having intercourse. These exercises are followed by those involving genital stimulation, which, in turn, are followed by a "teasing technique," when manipulative play and cessation of penile stimulation are alternated. The purpose here is to demonstrate the lack of impairment in the erectile response of the male and to alleviate the fear that loss of erection will not be followed by its return.

Five-year follow-up data were reported for 40% of the sample. For the 32 men with primary erectile dysfunction, the initial success rate was 59%. Five-year evaluations of 7 men revealed no return of the erectile problem. The initial success rate for 213 men with secondary erectile dysfunction was 74%. Follow-up data on 90 men indicated that 89% did not experience a return of the dysfunction.

Several modifications of the Masters and Johnson program have been described. In one, couples were treated once a week for 15 weeks (Lobitz and LoPiccolo, 1972). Patients were asked to complete daily record forms to monitor closely changes in their sexual behavior. Therapist role-modeling and patient role-playing with respect to sexual initiation, refusal, and emotional assertion were utilized so as to augment interpersonal sociosexual skills. Also, men with difficulties experiencing arousal with their partner during *coitus* were instructed to try to pair orgasm during *masturbation* with images or pictures of the partner. Four of six men were successfully treated.

Psychodynamically Oriented Couple Sex Therapy

An integration of psychodynamic and couple sex-therapy procedures has been extensively described by Kaplan (1974). Rather than viewing erectile dysfunction as a defense against the emergence of a specific anxiety, the alternative was offered that erectile dysfunction could be just one possible physiological concomitant of anxiety, irrespective of the source. Some men were seen as being excessively vulnerable to stress and as reacting with erectile difficulty, the stress not necessarily being sexual in nature. The treatment format combined the prescription of specific sexual assignments for the couple at home with psychotherapeutic and instructional interventions at the clinic. The assigned sexual experiences were those believed to promote erotic factors in the relationship and were similar to those prescribed by Masters and Johnson. During the clinic treatment sessions, psychodynamically oriented therapy was used. Sources of underlying anxiety and guilt were focused on, interpersonal difficulties between the members of the marital couple were dealt with, and a member of the marital dyad was counseled. While statistical data concerning the outcome of the treatment program were not presented in detail, the contention was that secondary erectile dysfunction had a good prognosis but that the prognosis for primary dysfunction was less favorable. Also, significant psychopathology or marital discord was found to hinder treatment progress, although cures could take place even in the context of a poor relationship or significant psychopathology.

Behavior Therapy

Several therapies have been derived from classic or operant conditioning as they relate to the sexual dysfunctions. Techniques have included systematic desensitization, *in vivo* desensitization, and assertion training. Systematic desensitization, pioneered by Wolpe (1958), requires the patient to imagine a series of sexual scenes while in a state of deep muscle relaxation. The scenes are ranked and presented in a graded order of increasing anxiety. New scenes are not presented until the patient has imagined the prior one without anxiety. The theory here is that there is an incompatibility between deep muscle relaxation and anxiety, and thus, the patient learns to experience the scenes without anxiety. Anxiety is seen as incompatible with erection. It is hoped that changes during therapy sessions will generalize to actual interpersonal sexual behaviors.

A treatment and follow-up study was reported where muscle relaxation was enhanced by intravenous barbiturate administration (Friedman, 1968). After a treatment program averaging nine sessions, 8 of 10 men maintained a cure at one-year follow-up. Another study with systematic desensitization was originally designed to employ methohexitone-induced relaxation during twelve 15-minute sessions (Friedman and Lipsedge, 1971). However, during the course of target symptom removal by systematic desensitization, the clinicians sensed that about a quarter of the maladaptive behaviors were being sustained by psychodynamic factors. Then, the duration of each treatment session was prolonged to 45 minutes to permit concurrent psychotherapy. Of the 19 patients with psychogenic impotence, 75% were symptom-free or much improved at follow-up (six months to five years).

Contrast Treatment Mode and Control Group Studies

A few studies include a contrast or control group. One compared the relative efficacy of systematic desensitization and interpretive group therapy (Lazarus, 1961). Five men were treated for erectile problems, two receiving group desensitization and three interpretive group therapy. Both men in the desensitization group reported recovery, compared with none in the interpretive group.

Two dozen men with erectile dysfunction of at least six months' duration, not believed to be secondary to a conflict in their nonsexual relationship, were reported by Kockott *et al.* (1975). Three groups of 8 men were matched for age, for primary or secondary erectile dysfunction, and on a neuroticism score. The first group received 14 sessions of systematic desensitization, and the second "routine therapy," which consisted of medication and "standard advice." Patients were seen four times over a three- or five-week period. The third group was placed on a waiting list for 15 weeks.

Measures at outcome included penile plethysmographic measurement of erection during the presentation of sexual situations and a subjective index of anxiety concerning coital situations described on audiotape. Clinical ratings of successful intercourse were also included. The patients in the desensitization group rated sexual feelings and sexual situations as being associated with less anxiety. Erection capacity tended to increase for both the desensitization and the routine therapy groups, but it decreased for the waiting-list group. Two patients were rated as cured and one was rated as improved in both the desensitization and the routine therapy groups, whereas one patient was rated as cured and seven were rated as unimproved in the waiting-list group. Subsequent to this study, 12 of the previous failures were treated by the same investigators, using a modified Masters and Johnson program. Now, 8 of the 12 were rated as cured or improved.

A study comparing systematic desensitization, psychoanalytically oriented group therapy, and a no-treatment control group was reported by Obler (1973). There were nine men in each of the three conditions. Unfortunately, the problems included secondary impotence, premature ejaculation, and ejaculatory incompetence, and the outcome data were not divided according to initial symptom. Furthermore, treatment effects were confounded in that the systematic desensitization group also received assertiveness training. The above notwithstanding, the systematic desensitization group reported superior gains, gains that remained stable over a 1½ year period.

One group study of systematic desensitization for secondary erectile dysfunction was that of Auerbach and Kilmann (1977): 16 men were assigned to either a group desensitization format or a no-treatment control group. The systematic desensitization group received 15 sessions of 45 minutes' relaxation plus a common hierarchy of sexual scenes, while the control group received 15 sessions of relaxation only. Both groups were told to expect improvement. Those receiving systematic desensitization had significantly more positive changes than the relaxation-only subjects. They also reported greater satisfaction with the nonsexual aspects of their relationship, gains that were maintained at the three-month follow-up.

Ansari (1976) used chemotherapy or a modified form of the Masters and Johnson technique to treat 65 men with a chief complaint of erectile dysfunction. A control group was not given any specific treatment. There were three subgroups of males: 21 had acute-onset dysfunction triggered by psychological or physical trauma; 23 had insidious-onset dysfunction due to long-term psychological or physical factors; and 21 had an insidious onset without discernible psychological or physical factors. The majority of men in Group 1 had become dysfunctional because of anxiety in sexual situations. In Group 2, dysfunction developed mainly because of the partner's low sexual responsivity or because of extramarital relationships. The distribution of subjects in the three treatment groups was not random. Some men were not assigned to the Masters and Johnson technique because they were single or because their partners were unwilling to participate. Subjects attended the outpatient clinic for six to eight months, being seen for a total of 12–14 sessions. The chemotherapy patients received oxazepam, an antianxiety drug. The Masters and Johnson technique was modified to involve only one therapist with the patients given homework assignments. The no-treatment control group attended the clinic for the same length of time and had history taking, physical examinations, and laboratory workups.

Fifty-five men completed treatment. The follow-up period was eight months. There was no significant difference in the outcome between treated and control subjects. However, the rate of recovery appeared to be related to clinical category. Subjects in Groups 1 and 2 showed a significantly better recovery rate than those in Group 3. The slightly higher rate of recovery seen in the controls was interpreted as being due to the higher number of Group 1 cases in this category. At the eight-month follow-up, there were more relapses in Groups 2 and 3. Age was not related to rate of recovery, whereas longer duration of dysfunction was associated with a poorer outcome.

Of additional interest here is that the Group 3 subjects appeared to differ from the other two in that they had an insidious decline in their sexual potency without discernible etiological factors and, from the beginning of their sex life, had shown a rather low sex drive. Because of this, testosterone (T) levels were measured to see whether low T-levels might be responsible for this pattern. No group differences were found.

Biofeedback Training

Although penile erection is usually regarded as an involuntary reflex to erotic stimulation, there is evidence that nonpatient subjects have some voluntary control over the erectile response (Henson and Rubin, 1971; Laws and Rubin, 1969). College-age volunteers have demonstrated the ability to suppress or enhance erections by instructions alone (Rubin and Henson, 1975), and when subjects are provided immediate feedback concerning their level of arousal, control of erection improves (Rosen *et al.,* 1975).

The finding that voluntary facilitation of erection in nonpatient males can be enhanced via biofeedback suggests the possibility of using this technique in treatment. In a case study, a middle-aged male who had never achieved or maintained an erection in either heterosexual or homosexual experiences was described (Herman and Prewett, 1974). His penile response to both male and female erotic slides increased significantly during 16 sessions involving contingent feedback. Erections decreased when feedback was administered in a noncontingent manner. Interestingly, the increases and decreases in penile responsivity were parallelled by changes in ability to masturbate to orgasm, changes in masturbatory fantasy (to a more heterosexual orientation), and changes in sexual arousal outside of the laboratory setting.

A controlled study of biofeedback training involving six males who had experienced erectile dysfunction from 6 months to 10 years was made by Csillag (1976). Five were exclusively heterosexual. The comparison group was six men without sexual dysfunction. All men completed two sessions a day for four days. They were instructed to fantasize sexual situations and to attempt to achieve erection under various combinations of biofeedback accompanying visual erotic stimuli. The volunteer subjects without dysfunction showed greater initial changes in penile diameter, but the amount of daily diameter increase dropped as treatment progressed. By contrast, the subjects with erectile dysfunction showed minimal initial changes, but their daily changes in penile diameter increased during the treatment procedure. Three of the five heterosexual men, two of whom had unconsummated marriages, achieved adequate improvement in erectile function for sexual intercourse.

Less optimistic findings were reported by Reynolds (1980). Thirty men with erectile failure were studied under three biofeedback conditions. Members of the first group received continuous feedback of erection changes and were shown the erotic film segments after an increase in erection. The second group was also shown the erotic film after an erection increase but did not receive continuous feedback. The third group also saw the film segments, but not necessarily in response to fuller erections.

There was no difference between the groups at the completion of therapy or at one-month follow-up. Clinical improvement was "slight" for all subjects combined. While two-thirds reported "some" improvement, only one-quarter reported "considerable" or "complete" improvement.

Mechanotherapy

The "penile ring" was utilized in a study of 40 men. The ring is made of ebonite with five small metal plates on opposite inner surfaces. It opens on a swivel so that the penis, the scrotum, and the testicles are enclosed within it but hang freely below. A mild electric current is set up by the metal plates in contact with the moist, acid-containing skin. The 40 men were assigned in a crossover design to the electrically activated ring and a "placebo" ring incapable of producing an electric current. All men experienced phases of baseline, "active" ring, "placebo" ring, a treatment-free interval, and follow-up.

There were trends toward improvement with both the "active" and "placebo" ring, especially the "active," although statistical significance was not achieved. Improvement, when seen, was usually found in those males with secondary erectile failure. The investigator (Cooper, 1974) concluded that the beneficial effects may have been due to the "tourniquet effect" of constraining blood in the corpora (cf. Chapters 1, 2).

Hypnotherapy

In most research utilizing hypnotherapy for erectile dysfunction, treatment is confounded by the use of a variety of other techniques, including sex education, homework assignments, and depth psychotherapy. While there are several successful case studies, there are no control-group designs and no comparative studies with other treatments.

The hypnotherapeutic approach has been extensively described by Beigel (1971). He noted that decades earlier, Diethelm (1936) recommended hypnosis when "impotence is related to lack of self-confidence, based on feelings of general inadequacy, or body overconcern, or where patients were unable to deal with dynamic factors." Beigel emphasized that hypnosis should address the "total personality of whose insufficiency in one or several respects nonorganic impotence always is the expression." From information derived from waking sessions, material is obtained for use under the suggestibility of hypnosis. Sometimes, revelations occur during hypnosis, such as previously pre- or unconscious homosexual feelings, which may be interfering with heterosexual arousal. In-depth probing is combined with desensitization to aversive components of the heterosexual experience. Age regression may be used. The patient may be led under hypnosis through experiences in which nudity or sexuality produced fear, punishment, or guilt. The findings from these procedures are interpreted in ways that aid in undoing negative associations.

As for the differential diagnosis of psychogenic versus organic impotence, in addition to masturbation and morning erection criteria, Beigel suggested attempts to induce erection under hypnosis and, finally, anticipating Masters and Johnson's 1966 work, stressed that the male must not "work" at obtaining an erection but should "surrender completely to the sensory pleasures that he has learned to enjoy and to provoke and, when the erection develops, to act in accordance with his feelings."

Conclusion

Again, both treatments and results are varied. Better differential diagnosis of organic versus psychogenic causes may help to clarify and improve outcomes. So may more individually styled therapies. It is gratifying that the few controlled studies that exist are so contemporary. Scientism is replacing anecdotalism.

References

Ansari, J. (1976). Impotence: Prognosis (A controlled study). *British Journal of Psychiatry, 128*, 194–198.

Auerbach, R., and Kilmann, P. (1977). The effects of group systematic desensitization on secondary erectile failure. *Behavior Therapy, 8*, 330–339.

Beigel, H. (1971). The hypnotherapeutic approach to male impotence. *Journal of Sex Research, 7*, 168–176.

Bieber, I. (1974). The psychoanalytic treatment of sexual disorders. *Journal of Sex and Marital Therapy, 1*, 5–15.

Cooper, A. (1968). A factual study of male potency disorders. *British Journal of Psychiatry, 114*, 719–731.

Cooper, A. (1974). A blind evaluation of a penile ring—A sex aid for impotent males. *British Journal of Psychiatry, 124*, 402–406.

Csillag, E. (1976). Modification of penile erectile response. *Journal of Behavior Therapy and Experimental Psychiatry, 7*, 27–29.

Diethelm, O. (1936). *Treatment in Psychiatry*. New York: Macmillan.

Finkel, A., and Thompson, R. (1972). Alternatives to androgenic hormones in treating male impotency. *Geriatrics, 27*, 74–76.

Friedman, D. (1968). The treatment of impotence by brietal relaxation therapy. *Behavior Research and Therapy, 6*, 257–261.

Friedman, D., and Lipsedge, M. (1971). Treatment of phobic anxiety and psychogenic impotence by systematic desensitization employing methohexitone—induced relaxation. *British Journal of Psychiatry, 118*, 90–87.

Gill, H., and Temperlay, J. (1974). Time-limited marital treatment in a foursome. *British Journal of Medical Psychology, 47*, 153–162.

Goldberg, M. (1973). Selective impotence. *Medical Aspects of Human Sexuality*, August 13, p. 32.

Hastings, D. (1971). *A Doctor Speaks on Sexual Expression in Marriage* (2nd ed.). Boston: Little, Brown.

Henson, D., and Rubin, H. (1971). Voluntary control of eroticism. *Journal of Applied Behavior Analysis, 4*, 37–44.

Herman, S., and Prewett, M. (1974). An experimental analysis of feedback to increase sexual arousal. *Journal of Behavior Therapy and Experimental Psychiatry, 5*, 271–274.

Johnson, J. (1965a). Impotence and the limbic system. *British Journal of Psychiatry, 3*, 300–303.

Johnson, J. (1965b). Prognosis of disorders of sexual potency in the male. *Journal of Psychosomatic Research, 9*, 195–200.

Kaplan, H. (1974). *The New Sex Therapy*. New York: Bruner/Mazel.

Kockott, G., Dittman, F., and Nusselt, L. (1975). Systematic desensitization of erectile impotence: A controlled study. *Archives of Sexual Behavior, 4*, 493–500.

Laws, D., and Rubin, H. (1969). Instructional control of an autonomic sexual response. *Journal of Applied Behavior Analysis, 2*, 93–99.

Layman, W. (1972). Pseudo incest. *Comprehensive Psychiatry, 13*, 385–390.

Lazarus, A. (1961). Group therapy of phobic disorders by systematic desensitization. *Journal of Abnormal and Social Psychology, 63*, 504–510.

Lobitz, C., and LoPiccolo, J. (1972). New methods in the behavioral treatment of sexual dysfunction. *Journal of Behavioral Therapy and Experimental Psychiatry, 3*, 265–271.

Masters, W., and Johnson, V. (1970). *Human Sexual Inadequacy*. Boston: Little, Brown.

Obler, M. (1973). Systematic desensitization in sexual disorders. *Journal of Behavioral Therapy and Experimental Psychiatry, 4*, 93–101.

O'Connor, J., and Stern, L. (1972). Results of treatment in functional sexual disorders. *New York State Journal of Medicine, 72*, 1927–1934.

Proctor, R. (1973). Impotence as a symptom of depression. *North Carolina Medical Journal, 34*, 876–878.

Reynolds, B. (1977). Psychological treatment models and outcome results for erectile dysfunction: A critical review. *Psychological Bulletin, 84*, 1218–1238.

Reynolds, B. (1980). Biofeedback and facilitation of erection in men with erectile dysfunction. *Archives of Sexual Behavior, 9*, 101–114.

Rosen, R., Shapiro, D., and Schwartz, G. (1975). Voluntary control of penile tumescence. *Psychosomatic Medicine, 37*, 479–483.

Rubin, H., and Henson, D. (1975). Voluntary enhancement of penile erection. *Bulletin of the Psychonomic Society, 6*, 158–160.

Salzman, L. (1972). Psychotherapy with patients with sexual disorders. In M. Hammer (Ed.), *The Theory and Practice of Psychotherapy With Specific Disorders*. Springfield, Ill.: Charles C Thomas.

Tuthill, J. (1955). Impotence. *Lancet, 268*, 124–128.

Wolpe, J. (1958). *Psychotherapy by Reciprocal Inhibition*. Stanford, Calif.: Stanford University Press.

CHAPTER 10

Endocrine Therapy of Erectile Failure

RICHARD GREEN

The discovery of gonadal hormones, later called *sex steroids,* followed by gonadotropins and, finally, releasing factors, has ushered in an era of exalted speculation, enthusiastic experimentation, and modest findings. Here are described enthusiastic early reports, interim modulation, and contemporary sobriety.

Hormone supplementation has been a logical strategy based on the premise that deficient sexual functioning is a reflection of a deficiency in those hormones considered necessary for sexuality. Thus, in one study, 250 collaborating physicians gave 1000 patients testosterone in a drug called Afrodex® (Margolis and Lesley, 1966). Afrodex® is 5 mg nux vomica extract, 5 mg methyl testosterone, and 5 mg yohimbine hydrochloride. The age range of the men was 20–91 with most between 41 and 60. There was a significant difference in improvement from the first to the third week in those patients who did not drop out during that period. Those reporting "excellent" and "good" results increased from 25% (Week 1) to 39% (Week 2) to 56% (Week 3). The report, unhappily, includes no discussion of any controls used in the study, nor are details given of any medical evaluations.

Later, no less than 4000 cases of Afrodex® treatment were summarized by Margolis *et al.* (1967). Patients received the medication for up to 10 weeks. Again, no placebo group was used. The criteria of effectiveness were self-reports, with improvement rates increasing over the duration of treatment. About 20% reported "excellent" results, 25% "good" results, 30% "fair" results, and 20% "no" results. In spite of the absence of a placebo group, the authors concluded that "this mixture is of significant value in the treatment of impotence."

Double-blind crossover studies of Afrodex® were conducted by Miller (1968) and Sobotka (1969). Miller found Afrodex® to be at least 2 times more effective than placebo as measured by the number of reported erections and orgasms.

The Sobotka paper is more fully described here because more patients were studied and there were greater intervals between treatment modes so as to assess carry-over effects. Fifty men, aged 26–73, were studied who had experienced erectile failure for a minimum of six months. Each received drug or placebo for four weeks, followed by a four-week rest period, followed by four weeks with the alternate agent. A marked increase in the average number of erections and orgasms per week was found in association with Afrodex®. There was a carry-over of this effect through the four-week no-treatment period (here the effect was still double the pretreatment baseline). By contrast, after the placebo period, the number of erections and orgasms decreased and reverted to baseline. The increase in erections and orgasms on Afrodex® exceeded that on placebo by at least 3 times.

Enthusiasm for these reports is tempered by the absence of a distinction between psychogenic and organic etiologies, the lack of control groups in the larger studies, other studies' failing to confirm the positive effects of exogenous testosterone in men with normal testosterone levels, the potential hepatotoxicity of methyl testosterone, and the fact that Afrodex® is not listed in the current *Physician's Desk Reference.*

A few controlled behavioral and hormonal studies of testosterone administration exist. In one, treatment was assessed in men without clinical signs of androgen deficiency. The subjects were 29 males with a mean age of 56.5 years. The criteria for inclusion were a diagnosis of erectile failure, with the dysfunction persisting for at least one year and due to an unknown etiology; the regular availability of a female sexual partner; and a desire to have intercourse at least once a week (Benkert *et al.,* 1976).

The study lasted 20 weeks. During the first 2 weeks, all subjects received placebo in a single-blind mode. During the next 8 weeks, 13 men, selected at random, received testosterone undecanoate (TU), while the remaining men continued to receive placebo. This study phase was double-blind. Then, all the men received placebo on a single-blind basis for 2 weeks, followed by an 8-week observation period without medication. In addition to behavioral reports, blood samples were drawn for total testosterone (T), free T, sex-hormone-binding globulin (SHBG), luteinizing hormone (LH), and prolactin (PRL).

Of the 29 men, 5 showed a therapeutic effect after the first 2 weeks of placebo treatment. Because of the random assignment of subjects, 4 were then given further placebo, while the remaining 1 was receiving androgen. During the next 8 weeks, an additional 4 in the placebo group as well as 4 in the hormone group also showed a therapeutic effect. During the 2 following weeks of placebo treatment, 1 more in the placebo group and 3 more from the prior androgen group also showed a therapeutic effect. Thus, a therapeutic effect was noted in 17 of 29 men (59%). As for the effect on blood serum measures, administration of TU for 8 weeks decreased SHBG and tended to increase T (Benkert *et al.,* 1979).

An obviously important implication of this study is that in males without demonstrable signs of androgen deficiency, administration of a long-acting androgen has no greater effect than administration of placebo. The importance of a placebo in a double-blind study is evident in that nearly 60% of the patients, whether they received placebo or hormone, showed significant clinical improvement.

Testosterone is clearly helpful to *hypogonadal* men (Davidson *et al.*, 1979; Skakkebaek *et al.*, 1981). In the first study, six men, aged 32–65, two with primary gonadal failure, and four with secondary hypogonadism, were given testosterone enanthate (TE), in dosages of 100 mg and 400 mg, or placebo, once a month. The study was double-blind. Patients completed daily logs of sexual activity as well as a mood-rating scale. The measure for total erections, nocturnal erections, and coital frequency showed a dose–response curve to TE. There was no consistent relationship between mood state and androgen status.

In the second study, there were 12 hypogonadal men, 6 with *hyper*gonadotropic hypogonadism, mainly castrates, and 6 with *hypo*gonadotropic hypogonadism, mainly men with Kallman's syndrome. With these patients, the oral agent, testosterone undecanoate (TU) was given and a double-blind crossover design utilized. Diaries were kept for sexual activities, and energy was assessed by checklists. There were convincing and rapid responses to the androgen, with an increase in sexual functioning and a reduction in fatigability, anxiety, and tension.

The discovery of yet another link in the hypothalamic–pituitary–gonadal axis (releasing factors) inevitably led to the testing of luteinizing hormone releasing hormone (LHRH) effects on male sexual function. An early study reported increased erectile function in 7 of 7 men with hypogonadism (Mortimer *et al.*, 1974), and a double-blind study also suggested promise (Davies *et al.*, 1976). In the later study, 10 men with secondary erectile failure were given LHRH or placebo in a crossover design. Subjective measures of general sexual interest were slightly increased with LHRH.

A more definitive study (methodologically, if not in the clarity of results) keeps alive the therapeutic potential for LHRH (Evans and Distiller, 1979). In a balanced, double-blind, crossover design, six sexually functional, apparently endocrinologically normal young men were given either LHRH or placebo 10 min before a 40-min laboratory session in which they were exposed to visual erotic stimuli. Sexual arousal was assessed by degree of tumescence, and blood samples were assayed for LH, follicle-stimulating hormone (FSH), and T.

There was no correlation between basal hormonal levels and any behavioral index of sexual arousal. LHRH increased LH and FSH, but there was no change in T. Behaviorally, there was a tendency for the men to rate their level of sexual arousal as higher following LHRH. When they were instructed to masturbate to orgasm, there was also a tendency for the men to reach climax faster after LHRH. Further, there was a tendency for the men receiving LHRH to experience a greater degree of tumescence while watching the erotic stimuli. Thus, there was a small behavioral effect on normal males, suggesting that for hypogonadal males there could be a more substantial one. However, the picture for psychogenic erectile failure remains undeveloped.

Oxytocin has also been used in the treatment of erectile failure. The basis for its trial was heightened sexual activity in rabbits and fowl (Merlin and Kihlstrom, 1963). Forty-eight men, aged 20–63, were studied in a double-blind design. Excluded from study were 11 men "who showed a clear psycho-therapeutically workable conflict towards their partner." There was a tendency for drug patients to show more improvement during the first week. When some patients who "had suffered from a urogenital disease considered to be important for the development of impotence" were deleted from analysis *post hoc,* the trend reached statistical significance ($p < 0.05$). Age was not related to outcome, but there was a suggestion of more improvement for men with a shorter duration of erectile failure (Lindberg, 1972).

A compelling argument for searching for an endocrine etiology of erectile dysfunction was advanced recently in a study of 105 consecutive referrals (Spark *et al.,* 1980). The men ranged in age from 18 to 75. Only 5 had primary erectile failure. Serum T, LH, PRL, and the thyroid hormones, T_4 and T_3, were measured, as was LH response to LHRH. *More than one-third* (37%) showed evidence of hypothalamic–pituitary–gonadal axis abnormality. Serum T was abnormal in 36 patients. Four categories of endocrine dysfunction were defined: *hypo*gonadotropic hypogonadism (20 patients), *hyper*gonadotropic hypogonadism (7 patients), hyperprolactinemia (8 patients), and occult hyperthyroidism (4 patients).

In the first group, pituitary tumors were discovered in 12 of 20 men; 1 more had a hypothalamic glioma. Erectile function was restored in 18 of 19 men with injections of either testosterone enanthate (TE) or human chorionic gonadotropin (hCG). For the 7 patients with hypergonadotropic hypogonadism, TE resulted in a dramatic increase in libido and return of erectile function.

Patients with occult hyperthyroidism, after treatment with propylthiouracil, showed lowering of T_4 and T_3, a fall of T to normal levels, and restoration of erectile capacity. In these patients, though serum testosterone levels appear elevated, the elevation seems to be an artifact reflecting increased production of SHBG. Hyperthyroidism was also previously found to be associated with loss of libido (71%) and decreased potency (56%) by Kidd *et al.* (1979).

The eight patients with hyperprolactinemia were treated with the dopaminergic drug, bromocriptine. With this treatment serum prolactin (PRL) levels usually fall, and serum T usually rises. In 6 of the 8 patients, once PRL levels were normal, erectile function returned.

Another series of patients with pituitary tumors secreting excessive prolactin was also found to have erectile failure and low testosterone levels. Bromocriptine therapy restored erectile function in 19 of 25 patients, 15 of whom had acromegaly, 5 of whom had prolactin-secreting tumors, and 5 of whom had hyperprolactinemia of unknown etiology (Thorner and Besser, 1976). By contrast, testosterone alone when given to men with hyperprolactinemia is generally ineffective in restoring potency (Spark *et al.,* 1980).

Conclusion

There is a subsample of males with erectile dysfunction who can benefit from endocrine therapy. These are men with endocrinopathy demonstrated by comprehensive endocrinological evaluations. In the absence of demonstrable endocrinopathy, any beneficial effect of endocrine therapy appears to be a placebo response. Sophisticated methods of assessing endocrine function should be able to identify the treatable subgroup. From the research standpoint, much remains to be learned about the interaction between amines, peptides, and steroids and how they modulate sexuality. In the meantime, from the clinical standpoint, treatment guidelines are finally being developed.

References

Benkert, O., Horn, K., Prickardt, C., and Schmid, D. (1976). Sexual impotence: Studies of the hypothalamic-pituitary-thyroid axis and the effect of oral thyrotropin-releasing factor. *Archives of Sexual Behavior, 5,* 275–281.

Benkert, O., Witt, W., Adam, W., and Leitz, A. (1979). Effects of testosterone undecanoate on sexual potency and the hypothalamic pituitary gonadal axis of impotent males. *Archives of Sexual Behavior, 8,* 471–480.

Davidson, J., Camargo, C., and Smith, E. (1979). Effects of androgen on sexual behavior in hypogonadal men. *Journal of Clinical Endocrinology and Metabolism, 48,* 955–958.

Davies, T., Mountjoy, C., Gomes-Pan, A., Watson, M., Hanker, J., Besser, G., and Hall, R. (1976). A double-blind crossover trial of gonadotrophin releasing hormone (LHRH) in sexually impotent men. *Clinical Endocrinology, 5,* 601–607.

Evans, I., and Distiller, L. (1979). Effects of luteinizing hormone-releasing hormone on sexual arousal in normal men. *Archives of Sexual Behavior, 8,* 385–395.

Faglia, G., Travaglini, P., Ambrosi, B., Beck-Peccoz, P., Paracchi, A., Weber, G., Bara, R., Elli, R., and Spada, A. (1976). Some aspects of prolactin influence on gonadal function in humans. In P. Hubinot, M. L'Hermite, and C. Robyn (Eds.), *Progress in Reproductive Biology,* Vol. 2. Basel: Karger.

Kidd, G., Glass, A., and Vigersky, R. (1979). The hypothalamic-pituitary-testicular axis in thyrotoxicosis. *Journal of Clinical Endocrinology and Metabolism, 48,* 798–802.

Lindberg, L. (1972). The effect of Syntocinon® on patients suffering from impotence. *Pharmakopsychiat, 5,* 187–190.

Margolis, R., and Lesley, C. (1966). Review of studies of a mixture of nux vomica, yohimbine and methyl testosterone in the treatment of impotence. *Current Therapeutic Research, 8,* 280–284.

Margolis, R., Sangree, H., Prieto, P., Stein, L., and Chinn, S. (1967). Clinical studies on the use of Afrodex® in the treatment of impotence: Statistical summary of 4000 cases. *Current Therapeutic Research, 9,* 213–219.

Merlin, P., and Kihlstrom, J. (1963). Influence of oxytocin on sexual behavior in male rabbits. *Endocrinology, 73*, 433–435.

Miller, W. (1968). Afrodex® in the treatment of impotence: A double-blind crossover study. *Current Therapeutic Research, 10*, 354–359.

Mortimer, C., McNeilly, A., Fisher, R., Murray, M., and Besser, G. (1974). Gonadotrophin-releasing hormone therapy in hypogonadal males with hypothalamic or pituitary dysfunction. *British Medical Journal, 4*, 617–621.

Skakkebaek, N., Bancroft, J., Davidson, D., and Warner, P. (1981). Androgen replacement with oral testosterone undecanoate in hypogonadal men: A double blind controlled study. *Clinical Endocrinology, 14*, 49–61.

Sobotka, J. (1969). An evaluation of Afrodex® in the management of male impotence: A double-blind crossover study. *Current Therapeutic Research, 11*, 87–94.

Spark, R., White, R., and Connolly, P. (1980). Impotence is not always psychogenic. *Journal of the American Medical Association, 343*, 750–755.

Thorner, M., and Besser, G. (1976). Hyperprolactinemia and gonadal function: Results of bromocriptine treatment. In P. Crosignani and C. Robyn (Eds.), *Serano Symposia on Prolactin and Human Reproduction*. New York: Academic Press.

CHAPTER 11

Penile Dysfunctions due to Local Disorders

GORM WAGNER

Priapism

Priapism is defined as an involuntary, long-standing, painful erection with a block of blood flow through the cavernous bodies, but with free flow through the glans and the spongiose body. If untreated, it often leads to fibrosis of the erectile tissue (Hinman, 1960), thus preventing normal erectile function. The prognosis is sharply worsened when priapism persists for more than 72 hours. While there are correlational abnormalities associated with the condition, the true etiology is not known.

Neurogenic, vascular, neoplastic, and traumatic causes have been identified. Blood disorders, especially sickle-cell anemia, are considered causative (Diggs and Ching, 1934). There are reports on alcohol- and drug-induced priapism. Besides cases with an underlying disorder, some are considered idiopathic. It may occur at any age, even in children (Menzel, 1953).

A study of eight men who earlier had idiopathic priapism (Money and Hirsch, 1965) described their sexuality 3 to 11 years later. Seven were rendered permanently impotent, but all had retained their feelings of orgasm and the ability to have an ejaculation.

In a recent study of 18 postpriapism cases, Lund and Ebbehøj (1980) found that 11 had normal erectile function after the surgical procedure introduced by Ebbehøj (1975). They classified 12 cases as idiopathic and 3 as possibly due to alcohol abuse, while 2 were related to trauma and 1 to leukemia. After surgery, 11 were completely improved, and 3 others showed some improvement. Erectile function was evaluated 2–56 months after surgery. Three patients with erectile dysfunction were reoperated on, and the persistent anastomosis was closed, as described by Ebbehøj and Wagner (1979). Figure 58, Chapter 12, demonstrates the simple surgical procedure advocated for priapism.

Abnormal Leakage(s) from the Corpus Cavernosum

Erectile dysfunction was described in three bulls by Ashdown and Gilanpour (1974). By careful postmortem studies, they discovered abnormal anastomoses between the cavernous bodies and the venous drainage system. In vascular casts, they demonstrated the phenomenon and assumed that these abnormal anastomoses were the cause for the erectile failure that the bulls had shown when trying to mate. Since then, other similar cases have been seen. Development and maintenance of a high pressure in the cavernous bodies are essential to erection, and it is obvious that a regulatory system of the outlet is necessary in this hydraulic system. This necessity helps explain the erectile dysfunction in some cases of surgically induced anastomosis between cavernous and spongiose bodies originally performed to relieve priapism.

In addition to this iatrogenic erectile dysfunction, other naturally occurring cases have been described (Ebbehøj and Wagner, 1979). In a congenital case, the patient may report that he had observed that his erection appeared to be different from that of other boys since his early teens. Others are not fully aware of their lack of rigidity until their early 20s. The penis responds rapidly with visual sexual stimulation, and a full tumescence is achieved. However, there is not sufficient rigidity to allow for normal vaginal penetration. In other cases, some rigidity is obtained, soon lost, reobtained, and then lost again.

The pathology may be a single or several perforations at the tip of the cavernous body, or it may exist as one or several large veins perforating the tunica albuginea. In some men, it may occur after several years of normal function and

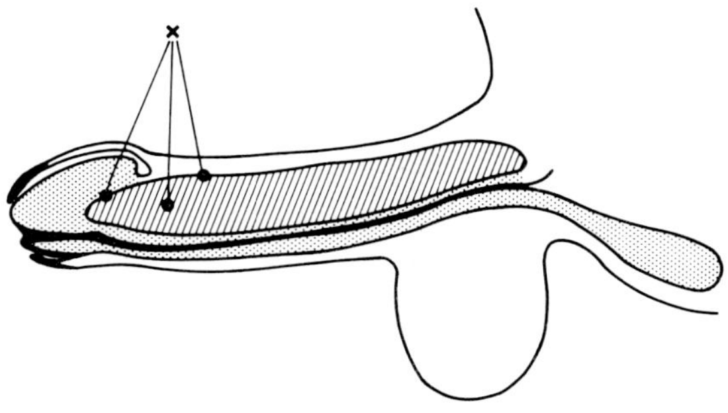

Figure 50. Schematic drawing of the penis with the most common localizations of fistulas or abnormal venous drainages from the cavernous bodies.

may be due to a slight burst of the tunica albuginea, even with the formation of a hemangioma (Figure 50).

The diagnosis can be made by exclusion of arterial insufficiency, by the existence of an increase in xenon washout during sexual stimulation, and by localization of the defect by infusion cavernosography combined with sexual stimulation. The surgical procedure is described in Chapter 12.

Peyronie's Disease

Peyronie's disease, or plastic induration of the penis, is a disease that may occur at any time in adult life, but most commonly in the fifth and sixth decades. It was originally described in 1743 by François de la Peyronie. The initial symptom may be pain with erection or bending of the penis, most pronounced during erection. It impairs vaginal intercourse.

A careful history and a careful palpation of the shaft of the penis may reveal the disease. One or more hard plaques may be felt, related to the tunica albuginea. It may occur on the dorsal, lateral, or ventral surface of the sheath, but always deep to the vessels and nerves. Any size can be found. The etiology is unknown, but it may sometimes be seen in conjunction with osteoarthritis or palmar fibromatosis. The plaques exhibit fibroblastic proliferation and, in rare cases, ossification.

The prognosis is difficult to state, as many patients experience spontaneous regression. In severe cases, a true erectile dysfunction develops and may be characterized by full erection of part of the shaft while the affected area does not increase in volume. On palpation, it feels as though a joint were inserted in the penis.

Treatment quite often does not help the patient. The numerous treatments suggested through the years include irradiation, surgery, vitamin E, or local cortisone injections. In a recent review, Palomar *et al.* (1980) concluded that the surgical implantation of a dermal graft is advisable only in young patients who have a small plaque and who are not impotent. They recommended that a penile prosthesis be inserted in elderly patients who have larger plaques and who are impotent. The incidence of Peyronie's disease among impotent males is not known, as the disease quite often is not recognized unless a cavernosogram is performed.

It does not seem logical to perform excision and grafting in a patient with no erectile failure unless there is bending of the penis. For the latter, a simpler technique is preferable (see the following section). It has been suggested that erectile failure in some cases of Peyronie's disease may be caused by abnormal drainage from the cavernous body, as can be visualized by dynamic infusion cavernosography (Ebbehøj, 1980).

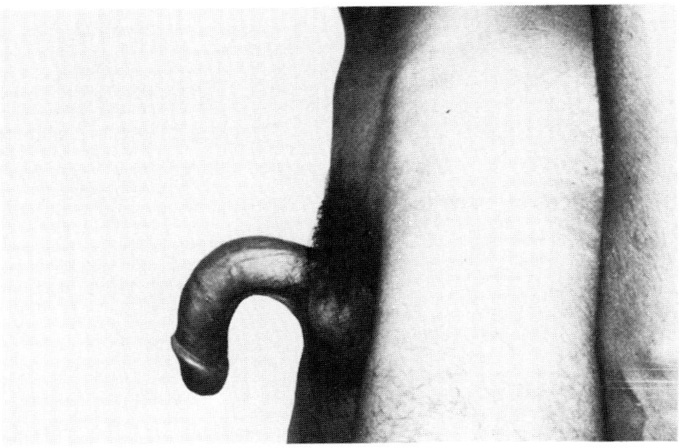

Figure 51. Lateral view of the erect penis in a 19-year-old man whose penis bends only when erect (a condition known as *Krummerik*). Photo taken by patient.

Bending of the Erect Penis

A patient who complains of bending of the penis during erection often may be unable to effect vaginal penetration. Peyronie's disease should be ruled out by palpation, as a plaque may be the cause of the disorder. Nothing else will be found to be abnormal. Sex drive, rigidity, ejaculation, and orgasm are normal. If the patient is unable to produce an erection in the office, he should be asked to do so at home and to arrange to have a photo taken so the degree of bending can be evaluated (Figure 51). If treatment is necessary it should be surgical, involving the tunica albuginea. The simplest procedure is to make folds of the tunica on the convex surface, when bent, and to suture these transversely placed folds to make a tuck. This procedure makes incisions in the tunica unnecessary (Ebbehøj, 1980).

Conclusion

The simple surgical treatment of priapism sometimes leads to erectile dysfunction because of an induced fistula. Also, fistulas may be congenital as well as acquired. Peyronie's disease should be ruled out by careful palpation, and erectile dysfunction due to a bent penis should be diagnosed by careful history taking.

References

Ashdown, R. R., and Gilanpour, H. (1974). Venous drainage of the corpus cavernosum in impotent and normal bulls. *Journal of Anatomy, 117*, 159–167.

Diggs, L. W., and Ching, R. E. (1934). Pathology of sickle cell anemia. *Southern Medical Journal, 27*, 839–846.

Ebbehøj, J. (1975). A new operation for priapism. *Scandinavian Journal of Plastic and Reconstructive Surgery, 8*, 241–242.

Ebbehøj, J. (1980). Presented at the *Second International Conference on Vasculogenic Impotence*, Monaco, Oct. 6–10.

Ebbehøj, J., and Wagner, G. (1979). Insufficient penile erection due to abnormal drainage of cavernous bodies. *Urology, 13*, 507–510.

Hinman, F., Jr. (1960). Priapism: Reasons for failure of therapy. *The Journal of Urology, 83*, 420–428.

Lund, K., and Ebbehøj, J. (1980). Results of glando-cavernous anastomosis in 18 cases of priapism. *Scandinavian Journal of Plastic and Reconstructive Surgery, 14*, 269–272.

Menzel, E. (1953). Der Priapismus beim Kinde. *Zentralblatt für Chirurgie, 78*, 89–92.

Money, J., and Hirsch, S. (1965). After priapism: Orgasm retained, erection lost. *The Journal of Urology, 94*, 152–157.

Palomar, J. M., Halikiopoulos, H., and Thomas, R. (1980). Evaluation of surgical management of Peyronie's disease. *Journal of Urology, 123*, 680–682.

CHAPTER 12

Surgical Treatment of Erectile Failure

GORM WAGNER

With erectile dysfunction, many patients hope for a quick, mechanical, nonpsychological treatment. This hope may be so pronounced that even after thorough examinations, as mentioned in earlier chapters, with no pathological findings, a patient will continue to express reluctance about sex therapy. Surgeons experienced with penile surgery know the pressure frequently exerted on them. Some men may demand "any kind of operation" that may give some hope of penile rigidity.

During the last decade three parallel developments have emerged in penile surgery:

1. Implantable prostheses (solid or inflatable)
2. Corrective surgery on the arterial supply
3. Corrective surgery on drainage failures

The history of surgical treatment of erectile failure dates back to the start of this century, and many different types of surgery have been advocated (Gee, 1975). Although the results are difficult to evaluate from the original papers, and follow-up studies are almost nonexistent, some of the surgical procedures on the deep dorsal vein may have been helpful to some patients. That patients were not carefully selected in all cases can be demonstrated by the authoritarian statement by the American urologist Lydston in 1908:

> The objection to operative measures based on a diagnosis of psychic impotence is absurd. The patient wants relief, not a psychic diagnosis. Scientific reasoning and psychopathic diagnoses fall to the ground before the absolute of a flaccid penis in a physiological emergency. (cited by Gee, 1975, p. 401)

Today's indications for performing surgery differ, and general indications cannot be given as they depend on a total evaluation of the particular patient. His basic disorder, motivation, psychological state, and age all have to be considered. The preoperative investigations for penile implants differ from those where an arterial or venous correction may be performed.

Penile Implants

Some surgeons accept cases for implants where psychotherapy and sexual counseling (Bias *et al.* 1975), as well as androgen therapy (Small *et al.* 1975), have been tried without success. Others accept only nonpsychogenic cases for implants (Debled, 1977; Subrini, 1980). In some clinics, a nocturnal penile tumescence (NPT) evaluation (see Chapter 8, p. 104) is required. Others, like Gee *et al.* (1974), suggest delaying a decision until comprehensive psychiatric evaluation is conducted. They advocate psychiatric consultation if there is doubt about the patient's motivation or a question of psychosis. The finding that patients who have made little attempt to try other means of sexual gratification in overcoming

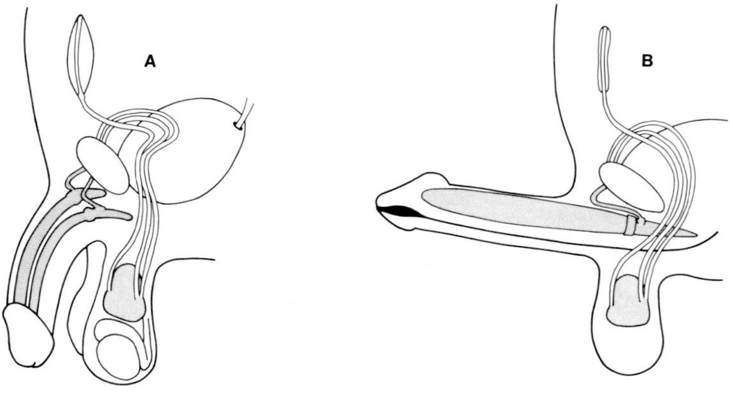

Figure 52. Scott inflatable prosthesis. The implanted prosthesis consists of a reservoir containing a radiopaque solution (A), silicone tubes, a bulb with pumping mechanism, and two silicone cylinders that can be filled with the liquid from the reservoir via the pump (B). The surgical technique needed to implant this prosthesis is obviously more sophisticated and extensive than for the cavernosus implants. The reservoir is placed in the prevesical space and the pump low in the scrotum outside the tunica vaginalis (for details, see Furlow, 1976). The advantage of a reconstructed physiological erectile appearance is obvious as is the appearance in the flaccid state. The specific advantage of this prosthesis is emphasized in the treatment of diabetics, who at a later stage may encounter neurogenic bladder problems with the need for cystoscopy and possible vesical neck surgery. This prosthesis may permit such urological investigations.

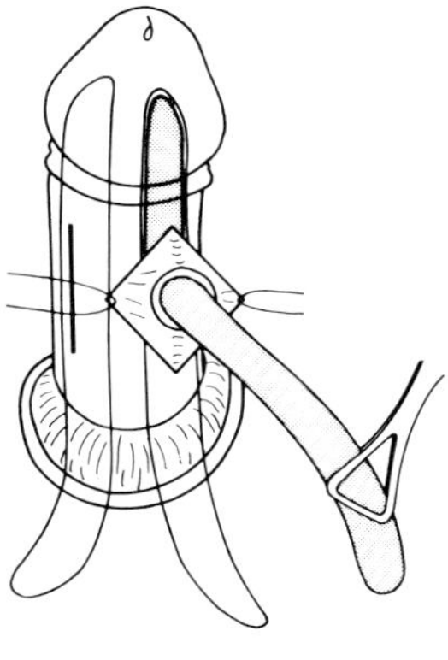

Figure 53. The Subrini prosthesis (Silastic® penile implant) consists of a firm and a soft silicone elastomer. The distal part is firm and the proximal more soft to contribute to a cushion effect and also to allow for bending the penis. These prostheses exist in diameters of 10 and 11 mm but only in one length. The surgeon has to cut the prosthesis to the proper length during the operation. The figure shows the shaft of the penis exposed; the right prosthesis is being placed after dilatation of the cavernous tissue through a lateral incision of the tunica albuginea. The conical end of the rod has to be well placed under the glans penis. (Reproduced by permission of the Dow Corning Corporation, the owner of the copyright.)

the erectile failure are poor candidates for implants points to the importance of careful screening of the motives and attitudes of the patient and his partner. Gee *et al.* suggested that this

> should include questions on 1) the degree of sexual activity before the patient became impotent, 2) specific means of sexual gratification attempted since impotence and 3) the importance to each partner of being able to have intercourse.

The use of the Minnesota Multiphasic Personality Inventory (MMPI) has been advocated (Furlow, 1976, 1978a) along with other psychological evaluations. Further, a preoperative discussion and demonstration of the implant device and its function are conducted, with both the patient and the partner present. Partner acceptance is taken into consideration.

The currently most widely used protheses are of two types: (1) paired silicon rods (Pearman, 1972; Subrini, 1973; Small *et al.,* 1975; Finney, 1977) and (2) inflatable (Scott *et al.,* 1973). Figures 52–55 demonstrate the different types of prostheses and the most common surgical techniques for their implantation.

During the first years of experience with implantation of the inflatable prothesis, more complications were reported than later (Furlow, 1976, 1978a). The better results are ascribed partly to the increased experience of the surgeons and partly to technical sophistication in instrumentation. The mechanical complications of the inflatable device were about 25%. In all cases, they have been correctable by a renewed, often minor, surgical intervention. Because of a change in product design, the failure rate has dropped to about 10%. The last 20 patients of a series of 103 patients had no complications (Furlow, 1978b).

Two main groups of patients, one postprostatectomy and the other diabetic, contributed 60% of the cases reported by Furlow (1978a). The most severe acute complication is infection, which, once started, eventually proceeds along the pathways made by the surgical procedure. This infection may necessitate removal of the prosthesis. The overall functional success is above 90%. Approximately 700 patients have now been operated on at the Mayo Clinic, which has reduced the complication rate to 6% with the intrapubic approach to insertion of the inflatable prosthesis (Furlow, 1980). Reports on longevity remain to be published. The cost of the inflatable prosthesis and the longer hospital stay with a major operation are two disadvantages of this device. However, the physiological appearance and function of the prosthesis is a major advantage (Wood and Rose, 1978).

A follow-up study of 175 men with the inflatable prosthesis, along with their

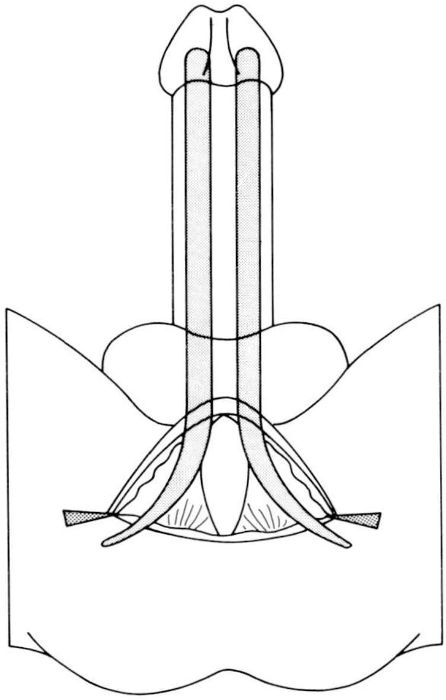

Figure 54. The Small-Carrion prosthesis shown inserted. The proximal portion of the prosthesis is curved to fit the crus of the cavernous body and is made of solid medical-grade silicone. The rest of the rod consists of a medical-grade silicone exterior with a silicone sponge interior. The prosthesis is available in four lengths (12, 13.3, 14.5, and 15.8 cm) and in 9- or 11-mm diameter. Usually, the prostheses are placed through a perineal surgical approach. The insertion takes place after identification of the crus penis, into which the incision is made. Then, dilatation with Hegar's dilators is done to the very tip of the cavernous body to ensure that the glans does not flex over the end of the rod.

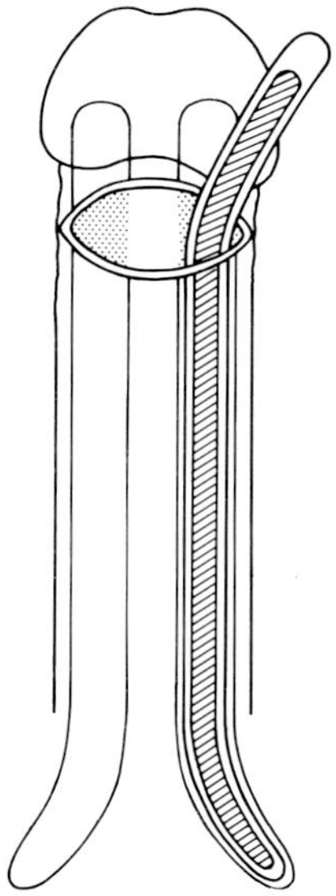

Figure 55. The Jonas prosthesis is made of silicon rubber; an area of its tip has lower resistance. In the silicone rubber, 10 silver wires of 0.6-mm diameter are imbedded to abolish the back force of the silicon rubber. Thus, tension, especially in the area of the crura, can be avoided. The prosthesis is available in six lengths (from 17 to 22 cm) and in 9.5- and 11-mm diameter. The dorsal incision at the distal end of the corpus cavernosum is advocated in order to achieve the best dilatation and placement of the distal part of the device.

sexual partners, was carried out by Gerstenberger *et al.* (1979). Half of the men were "very satisfied" with the result of the procedure, as were about half of their partners. Another quarter of both groups were "fairly satisfied." Eleven had been operated on for what was considered psychogenic impotence.

The rod implants are surgically easier to place and require only a few days' hospital stay. However, one major disadvantage is the constant semierection, which may be noticeable. In the first 110 cases operated on by Subrini (1980), the largest group of patients (39%) had arterial lesions at different locations; 29% were classified as neurogenic dysfunctions (postcolectomy, paraplegy, and diabetes); and another group (28%) had local fibrotic conditions (Peyronie's disease and postpriapism). There were 4 cases of rod extrusion. With one of these patients, replacement did not succeed. Extrusion occurred around the area of the urethral orifice. Another 4 cases were complicated by fracture of the rod. In these cases, the insertion of two replacement rods in another operation was successful. No infections were reported.

In 66% of the cases operated on, additional physiological tumescence occurred around the rods during sexual arousal. Of these men, 78% were satisfied with intercourse when questioned at follow-up more than four months after surgery. When no additional physiological erection occurred, only 44% were satisfied. Further, only 25% of the spouses were satisfied in this latter group. Subrini estimated that it takes about six months for the patient to feel that the implant is completely integrated, physically and psychologically. To the question "Are you globally satisfied having been operated upon?" 87% of the patients and 67% of the partners answered, "Yes."

Implantation of the Pearman prosthesis (a silicone rod type) has most recently been reported by Bias *et al.* (1975), who operated on 28 patients. Surgical complications occurred in one-third. Two instances of a fractured rod during intercourse were reported by the same man. Another man had breakage of the implant, and migration of the rod occurred in two others.

The Small-Carrion penile prosthesis and its surgical outcome are described in 19 patients by Gee *et al.* (1974); in 41 patients by Small *et al.* (1975); and in 20 patients by Debled (1977). Debled has had 100% success—no infections, no migration, and only a 24-hour hospital stay—but has not clarified the etiology of his patients.

Of the 19 patients operated on by Gee *et al.*, 15 reported success, and 3 had infections and subsequent removal of the rods; 1 patient was lost for follow-up. Gee *et al.* emphasized that the most satisfied patients are those who experienced a sudden impotence (due to trauma or surgery) in contrast to those with a chronic medical disease. These latter patients still have their basic disorder and are less likely to be satisfied with the results of the prothesis.

Excellent technical results in 37 of 41 patients were reported by Small *et al.* (1975): 12 were arteriosclerotic cases, 15 had spinal cord injury, and the rest included a variety of etiologies, among which were 2 psychogenic cases. Two patients had rod extrusion with severe wound infection. After complications were treated, only one complete failure resulted.

In 1978, Small reported on 160 cases with a follow-up period from 1 to 46 months. In these patients, who had had solid prostheses for two to three years, 152 reported excellent, 5 good, and 3 poor results. Although prosthesis surgery with the use of insert nonbiodegradable material is new, it seems clear that the need for such surgery is of some magnitude. Subrini (1980) estimated that between 4000 and 5000 men on a worldwide basis have been operated on yearly with implants. New devices are still being developed. Among these are the hinged type, as seen in Figure 55 (Jonas prosthesis) and the flexirod hinged type (Finney type). In the report of the first 100 cases (Finney *et al.,* 1980), 79 were operated on through a dorsal penile incision, while in the rest, the prosthesis was inserted through perineal incision. The authors have recommended the dorsal approach as giving rise to less postoperative pain. Also, they emphasized that the corpus cavernosum must be measured carefully during the operation and that the implant must be trimmed to the proper length, as they found that excessive length produced prolonged pain. The surgical complication rate was reported as 4%. The major groups of patients were diabetic (33%) or had "vascular diseases" (30%). Neurological causes comprised the major part of the remaining patients. In a combined three-hospital assessment from 1974–1979 in Pennsylvania (Malloy *et al.* 1980), the outcome of insertion of the inflatable implant (Scott prosthesis) was compared with that of a rigid-rod implant (Small-Carrion prosthesis): 105 patients with inflatable prosthesis were followed from 6 months to 4½ years, and a functional success rate of 93% was reported; in 45 patients with the rigid rod prosthesis, 88% satisfaction was found. Except for the advantages and disadvantages mentioned earlier in this chapter, the authors pointed to the problems that may occur when an endoscopic operation has to be performed in patients with solid implants. Attachment of an external continence device presents fewer problems with the solid implant. The authors suggested that a careful discussion has to be conducted with the patient as to the relative advantages and disadvantages of each device. They advocated that the patient actively participate in the selection process.

It seems obvious from the above that a careful selection and evaluation of the candidates for surgery are necessary, especially thorough information on both the patient and his partner. The diagnostic procedures used in previously published papers do not always seem to have diagnosed all cases correctly.

Female partners of 31 men who had received the Small-Carrion penile implant were evaluated by Kramarsky-Binkhorst (1978). Of the partners of 60 males who were initially contacted, 29 refused evaluation. One woman declined to be interviewed. The men were 31 to 78 years old. Of the 31 males who received prostheses, only 3 appeared to have erectile failure of unknown etiology. In the other cases, 18 were diabetic, 5 had undergone genitourinary tract surgery, 3 had generalized cardiovascular disease, 1 had an ileostomy, and 1 had experienced a stroke.

Almost half of the female partners actively sought a consultation with their partner's surgeon. Slightly less than half had been assured that there was no need to fear vaginal injury from the implant and that the implanted penis could not be impaired during intercourse. Many of the other women considered the plastic hard and possibly dangerous. One-third worried about their ability to "turn on" their male partners who required the prosthesis. There were a few cases of dyspareunia, or painful intercourse, but most were temporary. The author suggested that this dyspareunia may have been caused by unacknowledged fears and/or sexual abstinence. Common findings however, were: for 25%, refusal by the women to touch the partner's penis; for 25%, fear of harming the penis; for 25%, the impression that the penis was too short or too flexible. (By "too flexible" was meant that the phallus buckled at the tip, making penetration or continued thrusting difficult.)

Less than half (only 42%) of the women reported that the couple were totally satisfied with the results of the operation. Of special interest is that four women, although sexually active with their partners postoperatively, were unaware that the implant surgery had been performed until being interviewed.

It has been advised that in the context of preoperative and postoperative counseling, the woman might start Kegel exercises to strengthen the perineal musculature so that the shorter, thinner, more flexible penis may be more effectively contained (Karmasky-Binkhorst, 1978). Other reports describe sobering effects on postoperative marital adjustment. Stewart and Gerson (1976) described a case of successful prosthetic surgery with subsequent divorce, and Gee (1975) described a spouse who refused sexual intercourse after successful prosthesis implantation.

Arterial Surgery

Surgical treatment of aortoiliac thrombosis or aneurysms of the lower aorta may lead to erectile failure, or it may, if precaution is taken with the nerves during surgery, lead to improvement in a case of erectile dysfunction (May *et al.*, 1969). During operations for arterial insufficiency of the legs, extension of an iliac endarterectomy to include a reconstruction of an occluded internal iliac artery is possible. This will reestablish the the direct arterial blood flow to the penis and thereby restore erectile function.

If occlusions are placed more distally in the pudendal artery or in the penile artery, another approach to reestablish normal arterial flow and pressure conditions is necessary. Penile revascularization was introduced in the English-language literature by Michal *et al.* (1977); he had described it earlier in Czech

(Michal *et al.,* 1973). Under general anesthesia, the inferior epigastric artery is located (see Figure 56). The artery is isolated and shifted below the inguinal ligament and sutured into a cavernostomy. Of 21 patients (40–63 years old), all of whom had arteriographic diagnosis of arterial insufficiency, 13 had technically successful results with a patent anastomosis. Of these, 9 resumed normal sexual activity, and 3 developed priapism after surgery.

Most of these created anastomoses, as well as those in other studies with fewer patients, have occluded shortly after surgery. After one year, very few remained open. Only one surgeon claims to have a high success rate, with 90% initially successful and 75% still functional after one year (Ginestié, 1978).

Because of these poor results, Michal *et al.* (1980) have changed their surgical approach and now make an end-to-side anastomosis between the inferior epigastric artery and the dorsal penile artery on the same side (Figure 57). This procedure does not risk priapism, and the results seem to indicate a longer duration of functioning anastomoses, as after two years, 17 of 31 patients continue to have anastomoses that are functioning (Michal, personal communication).

Penile revascularization surgery must be regarded as being still in the early stage of development. Attention should be paid to the development of this field, as it seems that technical problems are largely responsible for the negative results. Refinement in diagnostics will also help in the selection of patients who are better candidates for this procedure, which is a more direct approach to arterial insufficiency and would seem to provide a more acceptable treatment for the patient and his partner. Arterial insufficiency in the functional state may also be based on true arteriovenous fistulas, as described by Zorgniotti *et al.* (1979).

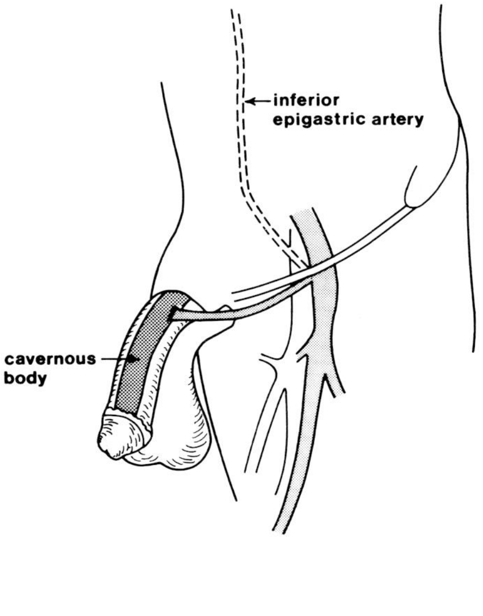

Figure 56. Schematic presentation of rearterialization operation, showing the move of the isolated inferior epigastric artery directly into the side of the ipsilateral cavernous body.

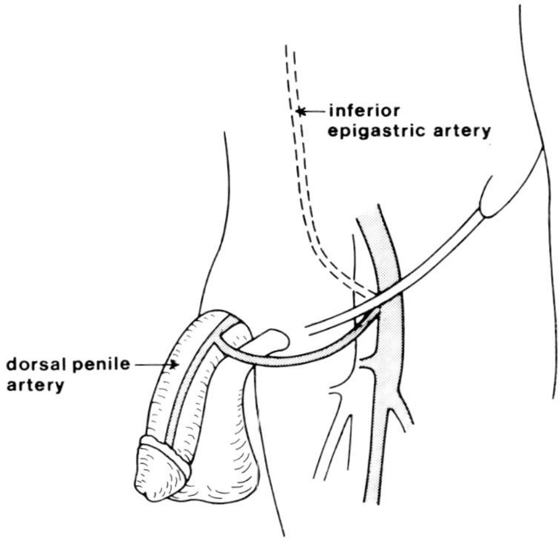

Figure 57. Schematic presentation of end-to-side anastomosis between the isolated and transposed inferior epigastric artery and the ipsilateral dorsal penile artery. Microvascular technique with the use of a microscope is necessary for the success of this procedure.

Corrective Surgery for Abnormal Drainage Conditions

Priapism is a disorder in which treatment may give rise to an iatrogenically induced erectile dysfunction. Throughout history, many surgical approaches have been tried. Some have been extensive and complicated. A recent very simple approach was given by Ebbehøj (1975) and is depicted in Figure 58. (For a description of priapism, see p. 149, Chapter 11.)

The induced fistula sometimes occludes and leaves the patient potent, but in

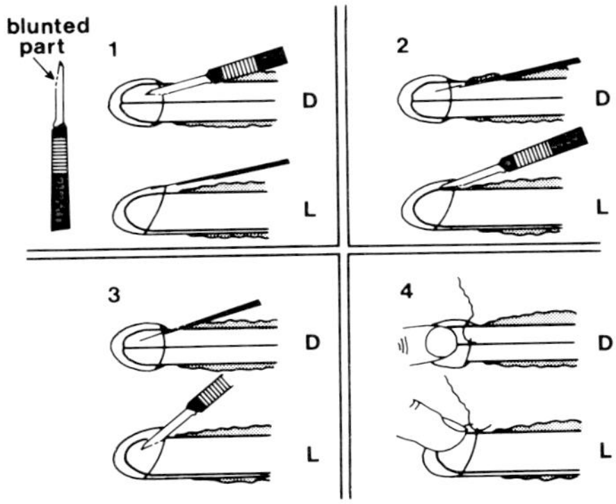

Figure 58. The Ebbehøj procedure for priapism (WHO list No. 5711). The surgery is done under local anesthesia. D: dorsal view. L: lateral view. The knife has to be blunted, except for the distal 5 mm. After insertion of the knife into the corona glandis (1), it is turned (2), and an incision is made in the tunica albuginea (3). This will allow free (arterial) blood to pass through the fistula into the glans. Then (4), the incision of the glans is closed by chrome catgut.

other cases, the persistence of the leakage from the cavernous spaces prevents erection. Flow measurement (p. 109) and infusion cavernosography (p. 114) will substantiate the diagnosis and locate the fistula. The closure is surgically simple. Under local anesthesia, an incision is made behind the corona. A dissection under the glans eventually leads to the area that is perforated. By injection of colored fluid into the cavernous body, the leakage is localized and the defect sutured (Ebbehøj and Wagner, 1979).

Abnormal leakage from the cavernous bodies may also occur as a cause for primary erectile failure, presumably as a congenital dysfunction (Ebbehøj and Wagner, 1979). Other cases may be acquired or may not become evident until a certain slight arterial insufficiency occurs. In cases where the leakage is well localized by cavernosography, the surgical intervention is simple and a good result seems to be permanent. To date, more than 30 patients have been operated on, some with iatrogenic fistulas, some with congenital fistulas, and some with acquired fistulas. Long-term follow-up studies of these patients remain to be conducted.

General Considerations

It would be incorrect to state that the patient with psychogenic erectile dysfunction should *never* have a prosthetic implant. Some psychogenic patients may not respond to psychotherapy and may still be very desirous of potency.

Until now, few patients who have had implants have been through the sophisticated vascular diagnostic procedures that have developed during the past few years. Thus, present diagnostic procedures may delineate those patients for whom a prosthesis rather than vascular surgery may be the treatment of choice.

Yet another consideration was noted in Chapter 5 (p. 70). The surgeon must avoid rushing the patient into the operating room immediately on demonstration of some forms of arterial insufficiency, as "spontaneous" remissions may take place, or drugs may be effective.

"Ideal" research cannot be conducted in this clinical situation. Here it would be necessary to conduct repeated arteriography in patients who improve clinically after a diagnostic procedure that demonstrated vascular insufficiency. The procedural risk must be considered. The clinical improvement of some patients immediately after pudendal arteriography indicates the need for a critical attitude toward the significance of an objective pathological finding. Because of these problems an international group of urologists and vascular surgeons have initiated cooperative studies that may shed light on these issues.

Another consideration is the emotional attitude toward a "foreign body" in an organ that does not function. There is also the adamant opposition by some clinicians to the insertion of a needle (however small) into the penis for diagnostic purposes. The medical profession must regard the penis as it does any other body organ in order that correct diagnosis and management may be conducted. To have a "device" placed in the dysfunctional penis is unacceptable to many. Yet hip-joint replacement does not evoke the same emotional response.

While most surgeons can learn the technique for implanting penile prostheses, they should be aware that this is just one part of patient management. Some patients and their partners may consider vascular surgical intervention more acceptable, since it corrects the hemodynamics of erection and is more "natural."

Experience shows that whether one or the other type of surgery is performed, it is vital that there be thorough discussion with the patient and his partner. It cannot be overemphasized that the couple should be followed for supportive counseling after surgery. The surgeon assuming responsibility for restoring (or creating) potency should carefully evaluate his or her professional role in these cases before launching on a surgical "adventure."

The development of an era of "wild surgery" should be avoided. We must prevent a jump from a psychotherapeutic ditch on one side of the road into a surgical ditch on the other. The middle road may well be the proper one to follow.

Conclusion

The surgical approaches to erectile failure are relatively new and exciting treatment innovations. These procedures offer considerable promise to men with otherwise untreatable forms of erectile failure. The implantable prostheses, some of which are relatively simple to introduce, may be used to correct a variety of defects producing erectile failure. Of special interest are the new vascular bypass procedures, as these more closely approximate normal physiological functions on the arterial side. However, they require more sophisticated differential diagnostic procedures. Also, the recent finding of abnormal drainage from the corpus cavernosum and its simple correction should be emphasized. Together, these approaches are at the frontier of the treatment of erectile failure, and the near future should bring provocative new techniques, studies, and findings.

References

Bias, H. I., Leverett, C. L., Parry, W. L., and Halverstadt, D. B. (1975). Implantable penile prostheses in impotent males. *Urology, 5*, 224–226.

Debled, G. (1977). La chirurgie de l'impuissance. *Acta Urologica Belgica, 45*, 349–353.

Ebbehøj, J. (1975). A new operation for priapism. *Scandinavian Journal of Plastic and Reconstructive Surgery, 8*, 241–242.

Ebbehøj, J., and Wagner, G. (1979). Insufficient penile erection due to abnormal drainage of cavernous bodies. *Urology, 13*, 507–510.

Finney, R. P. (1977). New hinged silicone penile implant. *Journal of Urology, 118*, 587–589.

Finney, R. P., Sharpe, J. R., and Sadlowski, R. W. (1980). Finney hinged penile implant: Experience with 100 cases. *Journal of Urology, 124*, 205–207.

Furlow, W. (1976). Surgical management of impotence using the inflatable penile prosthesis. *Mayo Clinic Proceedings, 51,* 325–328.
Furlow, W. (1978a). The current status of the inflatable penile prosthesis in the management of impotence: Mayo Clinic Experience Updated. *The Journal of Urology, 119,* 363–364.
Furlow, W. (1978b). Inflatable penile prosthesis: New device for cylinder insertion. *Urology, 12,* 447–449.
Furlow, W. (1980). Presented at the *Second International Conference on Vasculogenic Impotence,* Monaco, Oct. 6–10.
Gee, W. F. (1975). A history of surgical impotence. *Urology, 5,* 401–405.
Gee, W. F., McRoberts, J. W., Raney, J. O., and Ansell, J. S. (1974). The impotent patient: Surgical treatment with penile prosthesis and psychiatric evaluation. *The Journal of Urology, 111,* 41–43.
Gerstenberger, D., Osborne, D., and Furlow, W. (1979). Patient–partner satisfaction. *Urology, 14,* 583–587.
Ginestié, J. (1978). Results from arterio-cavernous revascularization. Paper presented at the *International Conference on Vasculogenic Impotence,* New York.
Karmasky-Binkhorst, S. (1978). Female partner perception of small-carrion implant. *Journal of Urology, 12*(5), 545–548.
Malloy, T. R., Wein, A. J., and Carpiniello, V. L. (1980). Comparison of the inflatable penile and the Small-Carrion prostheses in the surgical treatment of erectile impotence. *Journal of Urology, 123,* 678–679.
May, A. G., DeWeese, J. A., and Rob, C. G. (1969). Changes in sexual function following operation on the abdominal aorta. *Surgery, 65,* 41–47.
Michal, V., Kramář, R., Pospichal, J., and Hejhal, L. (1977). Arterial epigastricocavernous anastomosis for the treatment of sexual impotence. *World Journal of Surgery, 1,* 515–520.
Michal, V., Kramář, R., and Hejhal, L. (1980). Revascularization procedures of the cavernous bodies. In A. W. Zorgniotti and G. Rossi (Eds.), *Vasculogenic Impotence, Proceedings of the First International Conference on Corpus Cavernosum Revascularization.* Springfield, Ill.: Charles C Thomas, pp. 239–255.
Michal, V., Kramář, R., Pospichal, J., and Hejhal, L. (1973). Direct arterial anastomosis to the cavernous bodies of the penis in the treatment of erectile impotence (in Czech). *Rozhledy Chirurgia, 52,* 587.
Pearman, R. O. (1972). Insertion of a silastic penile prosthesis for the treatment of organic sexual impotence. *Journal of Urology, 107,* 802–806.
Scott, F. B., Bradley, W., and Timm, G. W. (1973). Management of erectile impotence. *Urology, 2,* 80–82.
Small, M. P. (1978). Small-Carrion prostheses: A report on 160 cases and review of the literature. *Journal of Urology, 119,* 365–368.
Small, M. P., Carrion, H. M., and Gordon, J. A. (1975). Small-Carrion penile prosthesis: New implant for management of impotence. *Urology, 5,* 479–486.
Stewart, T., and Gerson, S. (1976). Penile prosthesis: Psychologic factors. *Urology, 7,* 400–402.
Subrini, L. (1973). Surgical treatment with virile impotence: Intracavernous intubation. *Journal d'Urologie et Nephrologie, 79,* 647–653.
Subrini, L. P. (1980). Treatment of impotence using penile implants: Surgical, sexual, and psychological follow-up. In R. Forleo and W. Pasini (Eds.), *Medical Sexology,* The Third International Congress. Amsterdam: Elsevier, North Holland, pp. 629–635.
Wood, R. Y., and Rose, K. (1978). Penile implants for impotence. *American Journal of Nursing, 2,* 234–238.
Zorgniotti, A. W., Padula, G., and Rossi, G. (1979). Impotence caused by pudendal arteriovenous fistula. *Urology, 14,* 161–162.

Case Vignettes

Clinical Management and Outcome

A-2 Case Vignette

At the time of consultation, the patient was found to be in good general health. He candidly explained his sexual problems. External genitalia, genital reflexes, peripheral reflexes, and sensitivity were normal. There was a normal pulse and no bruits in the groin. Hemoglobin, sedimentation rate, creatinine, and glucose were normal. Testosterone, prolactin, luteinizing hormone (LH), and follicle-stimulating hormone (FSH) were also within normal limits.

The penile blood pressure index was 0.82 (at the low end of normal). Strain-gauge plethysmography with visual sexual stimulation revealed that the time to maximal tumescence was low for his age, and that no erection occurred. Blood flow (xenon washout) showed the following:

At rest: 3.6 ml/min/100g
During visual stimulation: 1.6 ml
Poststimulatory flow: 15.3 ml
Postocclusive flow: doubled from pretest values

The conclusion from these studies was normal venous regulation at stimulation with low postischemic flow.

Infusion cavernosography showed a slow washout in the flaccid state and a maximal intracavernous pressure at stimulation: 13 mm Hg. The conclusion from this study was that there was no abnormal drainage.

Arteriography (bilateral internal iliacs) showed stenosis of the proximal part of the right pudendal artery and bilateral occlusion in the distal part of the internal pudendals (Figure 45, Chapter 8).

The patient was told that his erectile failure was caused by arterial insufficiency, and he was informed of the possibility of arterial reconstructive surgery or a penile implant. He was asked to discuss these possibilities with his wife and to return after the decision. Three months later they decided on arterial surgery.

B-2 Case Vignette

At consultation, the patient was found to be of average intelligence, expensively clothed, and rather reticent, though providing precise answers to direct questions. He appeared pale. His heart rate and lungs were normal. There were no bruits in the groin. He was overweight by about 10 kg.

His testosterone, prolactin, FSH, LH, and thyroxine levels were normal, as were his blood sugar, creatinine, and hemoglobin. His sperm count was normal. His external genitalia and genital reflexes were normal.

Penile strain-gauge plethysmography and visual erotic stimulation were explained to him. During the first sequence, there was no tumescence. During the second, there was a normal tumescence phase of short duration with the development of full erection.

This finding was discussed, whereupon the patient eloquently (and seemingly with relief) described the pressure he felt about the infertility problem and the demands placed on him to function during his wife's periods of ovulation. He was referred back to the infertility clinic with the suggestion for couple psychotherapy.

Diagnosis: psychogenic erectile dysfunction, secondary to an infertility problem ("breeding syndrome").

C-2 Case Vignette

The therapist refused to discontinue Antabuse® and asked the patient to bring his wife to the next consultation. During that session, she declared that the sexual problems had been going on for years. She stated that she was disgusted with sexual intercourse with an inebriated husband and tried to refuse intercourse at these times. Sometimes, she was too frightened to refuse. Frequently, he was incapable of obtaining an erection, although he claimed to be very libidinous. Furthermore, she found that sexual problems were less important at the moment because of their generalized disagreement about "life." She said she did not find sexuality very attractive in such a situation.

During the next months, both partners attended the consultations. The work during these sessions was primarily directed at their overall communication and interaction and less at their sexuality. While they were informed about the present knowledge about sexual dysfunction, no specific sex therapy was started. One month later, he began work at a new job, where he functioned well. The couple's overall communication improved. Her sexual disgust was reduced, and his erectile capacity seemed better. At the time he left treatment, five months after beginning, he stated that they had sexual intercourse once a week, and though he did not have full erection, it was sufficient for intromission. By this time, he was being maintained without medication.

D-2 Case Vignette

Physical examination revealed a normal appearance and good general health. Genitalia and genital reflexes were normal. There was a palpable pulse and no bruits in the groin. Routine blood tests were normal. Plasma testosterone, LH, FSH, thyroxine, and glucose were also normal.

Penile blood pressure index (PBPI) was 0.49 (abnormally low). On this indication, arteriography was performed and showed total occlusion of the lowest 4 cm of the abdominal aorta and filling of apparently normal iliac arteries through lumbar and pelvic collaterals.

Diagnosis: external iliac steal syndrome due to occlusion of the aorta.

Vascular surgery with the implant of an aortoiliac trousers' graft prosthesis relieved symptoms in the legs, and the patient regained the ability to maintain erection during coitus. At follow-up, PBPI was 0.88 (normal).

E-2 Case Vignette

PBPI was 0.82 (low normal). There was a sluggish reaction to visual erotic stimulation, and there was no penile response to vibration. Cystometry revealed a neurogenic bladder with 50 ml residual urine. Achilles tendon reflexes were absent. Penile blood flow was normal at rest. With stimulation, a slight increase was noted. There was only a slight increase in postocclusive flow.

Infusion cavernosography revealed no abnormal leakages, but the outflow did not stop during visual sexual stimulation. There was only a modest increase in intracavernous pressure.

Diagnosis: erectile dysfunction due to impaired neural regulation, secondary to diabetes mellitus.

The possibility of a prosthesis was discussed with the patient, but he was repulsed by the idea. It was suggested that he and his wife return for further discussion and that they consider sex counseling.

F-2 Case Vignette

Physical examination revealed a healthy young man. He explained that he became normally aroused and had a fast penile response to sexual stimuli. He had morning erections, masturbated, and had no ejaculatory disorders. His main problem was lack of rigidity. The angle of the penis when stimulated was about −45 degrees from the horizontal.

Cavernosography was performed, and free flow was seen from the cavernous body into the glans. Surgery was performed, and the glans was separated from the tunica albuginea. A 2 by 5 mm opening into the cavernous tissue was localized close to the tip of the left cavernous body. This was sutured. A week later, he had his first normal erection. At the two-year follow-up, he was married, had a child, and had no erectile difficulties.

G-2 Case Vignette

The patient appeared shy and reluctant to talk in precise terms about his erectile problems. There was no story of the exact circumstances immediately prior to the loss of erectile ability.

His sexual drive had always been modest, and he stated that he never masturbated. Morning erections still occurred but not with any pronounced rigidity. He felt ashamed of his inability to erect and mostly avoided direct questions. He declared that he was not able to be sexually aroused by viewing pornographic pictures and believed that visual stimulation would not be of any help in diagnosis.

Infusion cavernosography with visual sexual stimulation revealed leakage through a large vein that did not close during the examination. It was localized in the distal part of the dorsal surface of the cavernous body. During surgery, it was removed and found to contain scar tissue. A month later, he reported better erections with rigidity that could be maintained during intercourse.

H-2 Case Vignette

The patient was found to be slightly overweight, somewhat shy, but circumstantial in his explanations. He reported, in a detailed sex history, that he had been able to produce an erection that permitted vaginal intromission but with only one girlfriend whom he occasionally visited. Morning erections were described as better than induced erections. Occasionally, he experienced premature ejaculation.

With visual sexual stimulation, his penile response was slower than normal for his age (Figure 26). The PBPI was 1.1 (normal). Xenon flow revealed a low basal flow but no venous leakage. Infusion cavernosography showed a sluggish filling and a slow washout in the flaccid state. Bilateral arteriography was performed because of the suspicion of arterial insufficiency. The X-ray (Figure 44) showed bilateral lack of distal segments of the internal pudendal arteries with the development of accessory pudendal arteries with low flow. There was slowed filling of the penile arteries.

The patient was advised to take more time when attempting intercourse to allow for necessary stiffness prior to attempting intromission. He was also informed about penile implants but was advised not to consider this alternative until further experimentation with longer foreplay, particularly involving penile tactile stimulation.

I-2 Case Vignette

With visual erotic stimuli the patient had no penile response (Figure 26A). PBPI was in the low normal range. Blood flow studies were normal, and no abnormalities were found in the genitalia or the genital reflexes. Endocrine studies were normal. No abnormal leakage was found at infusion cavernosography. Bilateral arteriography showed normal penile arteries with normal filling time. He was diagnosed as having psychogenic erectile dysfunction and was referred for couple sex therapy.

Conclusion

RICHARD GREEN AND GORM WAGNER

As noted in the Preface, erectile function is an elemental, yet complex, issue for men, engaging the realms of procreation, recreation, and self-image. Recent years have witnessed increased recognition of the vital interface between sexual health or disease and general health or disease. This recognition is exemplified by the World Health Organization's 1975 definition of "sexual health": "Sexual health is the integration of the somatic, emotional, intellectual, and social aspects of sexual being, in ways that are positively enriching and that enhance personality, communication and love."

The past decade has witnessed remarkable advances related to sexual behavior in the basic sciences of physiology, endocrinology, neuroendocrinology, and psychoneuroendocrinology. Remarkable advances have also emerged from the clinical sciences of psychology and psychiatry, as well as general surgery and microsurgery.

Concomitantly, there has been a revolution in the recognition and candid discussion of sexual dysfunctions. There has been a revolution in the differential diagnosis of the sexual dysfunctions. And there has been a revolution in the treatment of the sexual dysfunctions.

We hope we have captured the excitement of this exploding frontier. We hope and expect that the contents of this book will soon be dated. We hope, however, that the spirit of inquiry, clinical intervention, and scientific appraisal of this elemental, yet complex, feature of men will not be dated.

If our optimism is well founded, a future work will reflect continuing clinical progress in what we noted in the Preface as "this unique set of human dimensions." But for now, we are confident and content that the clinical course of the next patient presenting in the consultation room with the complaint of "impotence" has been remarkably improved.

Index

Page numbers in boldface indicate subject is treated in illustrations and/or table.